# OTHER FAST FACTS BOOKS



**Fast Facts for the NEW NURSE PRACTITIONER:** What You Really Need to Know in a Nutshell, 2e (*Aktan*)

**Fast Facts for the ER NURSE:** Emergency Department Orientation in a Nutshell, 3e (*Buettner*)

**Fast Facts About GI AND LIVER DISEASES FOR NURSES:** What APRNs Need to Know in a Nutshell (*Chaney*)

**Fast Facts for the MEDICAL–SURGICAL NURSE:** Clinical Orientation in a Nutshell (*Ciocco*)

**Fast Facts for the NURSE PRECEPTOR:** Keys to Providing a Successful Preceptorship in a Nutshell (*Ciocco*)

**Fast Facts for the OPERATING ROOM NURSE:** An Orientation and Care Guide in a Nutshell (*Criscitelli*)

**Fast Facts for the ANTEPARTUM AND POSTPARTUM NURSE:** A Nursing Orientation and Care Guide in a Nutshell (*Davidson*)

**Fast Facts for the NEONATAL NURSE:** A Nursing Orientation and Care Guide in a Nutshell (*Davidson*)

**Fast Facts About PRESSURE ULCER CARE FOR NURSES:** How to Prevent, Detect, and Resolve Them in a Nutshell (*Dziedzic*)

**Fast Facts for the GERONTOLOGY NURSE:** A Nursing Care Guide in a Nutshell (*Eliopoulos*)

**Fast Facts for the LONG-TERM CARE NURSE:** What Nursing Home and Assisted Living Nurses Need to Know in a Nutshell (*Eliopoulos*)

**Fast Facts for the CLINICAL NURSE MANAGER:** Managing a Changing Workplace in a Nutshell, 2e (*Fry*)

**Fast Facts for EVIDENCE-BASED PRACTICE:** Implementing EBP in a Nutshell, 2e (*Godshall*)

**Fast Facts for Nurses About HOME INFUSION THERAPY:** The Expert's Best Practice Guide in a Nutshell (*Gorski*)

**Fast Facts About NURSING AND THE LAW:** Law for Nurses in a Nutshell (*Grant, Ballard*)

**Fast Facts for the L&D NURSE:** Labor & Delivery Orientation in a Nutshell, 2e (*Groll*)

**Fast Facts for the RADIOLOGY NURSE:** An Orientation and Nursing Care Guide in a Nutshell (*Grossman*)

**Fast Facts on ADOLESCENT HEALTH FOR NURSING AND HEALTH PROFESSIONALS:** A Care Guide in a Nutshell (*Herrman*)

**Fast Facts for the FAITH COMMUNITY NURSE:** Implementing FCN/Parish Nursing in a Nutshell (*Hickman*)

**Fast Facts for the CARDIAC SURGERY NURSE:** Caring for Cardiac Surgery Patients in a Nutshell, 2e (*Hodge*)

**Fast Facts About the NURSING PROFESSION:** Historical Perspectives in a Nutshell (*Hunt*)

**Fast Facts for the CLINICAL NURSING INSTRUCTOR:** Clinical Teaching in a Nutshell, 2e (*Kan, Stabler-Haas*)

**Fast Facts for the WOUND CARE NURSE:** Practical Wound Management in a Nutshell (*Kifer*)

**Fast Facts About EKGs FOR NURSES:** The Rules of Identifying EKGs in a Nutshell (*Landrum*)

**Fast Facts for the CRITICAL CARE NURSE:** Critical Care Nursing in a Nutshell (*Landrum*)

**Fast Facts for the TRAVEL NURSE:** Travel Nursing in a Nutshell (*Landrum*)

**Fast Facts for the SCHOOL NURSE:** School Nursing in a Nutshell, 2e (*Loschiavo*)

**Fast Facts About CURRICULUM DEVELOPMENT IN NURSING:** How to Develop & Evaluate Educational Programs in a Nutshell (*McCoy, Anema*)

**Fast Facts for DEMENTIA CARE:** What Nurses Need to Know in a Nutshell (*Miller*)

**Fast Facts for HEALTH PROMOTION IN NURSING:** Promoting Wellness in a Nutshell (*Miller*)

**Fast Facts for STROKE CARE NURSING:** An Expert Guide in a Nutshell (*Morrison*)

**Fast Facts for the MEDICAL OFFICE NURSE:** What You Really Need to Know in a Nutshell (*Richmeier*)

**Fast Facts for the PEDIATRIC NURSE:** An Orientation Guide in a Nutshell (*Rupert, Young*)

**Fast Facts About the GYNECOLOGICAL EXAM FOR NURSE PRACTITIONERS:** Conducting the GYN Exam in a Nutshell (*Secor, Fantasia*)

**Fast Facts for the STUDENT NURSE:** Nursing Student Success in a Nutshell (*Stabler-Haas*)

**Fast Facts for CAREER SUCCESS IN NURSING:** Making the Most of Mentoring in a Nutshell (*Vance*)

**Fast Facts for the TRIAGE NURSE:** An Orientation and Care Guide in a Nutshell (*Visser, Montejano, Grossman*)

**Fast Facts for DEVELOPING A NURSING ACADEMIC PORTFOLIO:** What You Really Need to Know in a Nutshell (*Wittmann-Price*)

**Fast Facts for the HOSPICE NURSE:** A Concise Guide to End-of-Life Care (*Wright*)

**Fast Facts for the CLASSROOM NURSING INSTRUCTOR:** Classroom Teaching in a Nutshell (*Yoder-Wise, Kowalski*)

## *Forthcoming FAST FACTS Books*

**Fast Facts About PTSD:** A Clinician's Guide to Post-Traumatic Stress Disorder in a Nutshell (*Adams*)

**Fast Facts on COMBATING NURSE BULLYING, INCIVILITY, AND WORKPLACE VIOLENCE:** What Nurses Need to Know in a Nutshell (*Ciocco*)

**Fast Facts for the OPERATING ROOM NURSE:** An Orientation and Care Guide in a Nutshell, 2e (*Criscitelli*)

**Fast Facts for TESTING AND EVALUATION IN NURSING:** Teaching Skills in a Nutshell (*Dusaj*)

**Fast Facts for the CLINICAL NURSING INSTRUCTOR:** Nursing Student Success in a Nutshell, 3e (*Kan, Stabler-Haas*)

**Fast Facts for the CRITICAL CARE NURSE:** Critical Care Nursing in a Nutshell, 2e (*Landrum*)

**Fast Facts About NURSING PATIENTS WITH MENTAL ILLNESS (MI):** What RNs, NPs, and New Psych Nurses Need to Know (*Marshall*)

**Fast Facts for CURRICULUM DEVELOPMENT IN NURSING:** How to Develop & Evaluate Educational Programs in a Nutshell, 2e (*McCoy, Anema*)

**Fast Facts About the GYNECOLOGIC EXAM:** A Professional Guide for NPs, PAs, and Midwives, 2e (*Secor, Fantasia*)

**Visit www.springerpub.com** to order.

# *FAST FACTS About* *the* **NURSING PROFESSION**

**Deborah Dolan Hunt, PhD, MS, RN,** is associate professor of nursing and chair of the master's program at the College of New Rochelle, New Rochelle, New York. She has spent most of her career in nursing education, initially in staff development and currently in an academic setting. She is currently serving as one of the coleads for the New York State Future of Nursing's Action Coalition in the Northern Metropolitan Region and is a member of the advisory board for the Advance Healthcare Network. Dr. Hunt is also a member of Community Board 10 in the Bronx and the chairperson of its health and human services committee. She is a fellow of the New York Academy of Medicine and an ambassador and merit reviewer for the Patient Centered Outcomes Research Institute. In addition, Dr. Hunt is a member of Sigma Theta Tau International Honor Society of Nursing and has received the Zeta Omega research award for her doctoral dissertation. She was also the Sigma Theta Tau Zeta Omega Scholar from 2010 to 2011. Her research interests concern nursing turnover, job satisfaction, leadership, patient outcomes, and new nurse transition. Dr. Hunt's scholarly pursuits and teaching specialties include nursing education, the history of nursing, medical–surgical nursing, and transcultural nursing. She is the author of *The New Nurse Educator, Second Edition* (Springer Publishing, 2018) and *The Nurse Professional: Leveraging Your Education for Transition Into Practice* (Springer Publishing, 2014). Dr. Hunt has published many articles and has presented locally, nationally, and globally.

# *FAST FACTS About* *the* NURSING PROFESSION

## Historical Perspectives in a Nutshell

Deborah Dolan Hunt, PhD, MS, RN

SPRINGER PUBLISHING COMPANY
NEW YORK

Springer Publishing Company, LLC
11 West 42nd Street
New York, NY 10036
www.springerpub.com

*Acquisitions Editor:* Margaret Zuccarini
*Senior Production Editor:* Kris Parrish
*Compositor:* Westchester Publishing Services

*ISBN:* 978-0-8261-3138-6
*e-book ISBN:* 978-0-8261-3139-3



**Library of Congress Cataloging-in-Publication Data**

Names: Hunt, Deborah Dolan.
Title: Fast facts about the nursing profession : historical perspectives in a nutshell / Deborah Dolan Hunt, editor.
Other titles: Fast facts (Springer Publishing Company)
Description: New York, NY : Springer Publishing Company, LLC, [2017] | Series: Fast facts | Includes bibliographical references.
Identifiers: LCCN 2016051760 | ISBN 9780826131386 (hard copy : alk. paper) | ISBN 9780826131393 (e-book)
Subjects: | MESH: History of Nursing | Education, Nursing—history
Classification: LCC RT51 | NLM WY 11.1 | DDC 610.73—dc23 LC record available at https://lccn.loc.gov/2016051760



Printed in the United States of America by Gasch Printing.

*This book is dedicated to Brian, Meaghan, and John, who are my inspiration and always at the center of my universe, and to my parents and sister, who have always supported my dreams.*

*I also dedicate this book to our nursing historians and to all the nurses, doctors, and other health care professionals past, present, and future, who have tirelessly worked to promote the health and well-being of all.*

*Finally, this book is dedicated to the memory of Dr. Jean Whelan (1949–2017), nurse historian and past president of the American Association for the History of Nursing (2014–2016).*

*"The life of the dead is placed in the memory of the living."*
*—Marcus Tullius Cicero*

# Contents

## Part II FLORENCE NIGHTINGALE AND BEYOND



## Part III NURSING PROFESSION IN THE 21ST CENTURY

# Contributors

**Deborah Dolan Hunt, PhD, MS, RN**

Associate Professor of Nursing
Chair of the Master's Program
College of New Rochelle
New Rochelle, New York

**Brigid Lusk, PhD, RN, FAAN**

Professor
College of Nursing
University of Illinois at Chicago
Chicago, Illinois

**Donna M. Nickitas, PhD, RN, NEA-BC, CNE, FAAN**

Professor
Executive Officer, Nursing PhD Program at the CUNY Graduate Center
Hunter-Bellevue School of Nursing
Hunter College
New York, New York

**Jean Whelan, PhD, RN***

Adjunct Associate Professor
University of Pennsylvania School of Nursing
Philadelphia, Pennsylvania

*Deceased.

# Foreword

This book is designed to introduce the historical, global, societal, and scientific events that have patterned and influenced today's health care system. An understanding of these events is pivotal for understanding how we practice nursing today.

Nursing is a dynamic, complex, and ever-changing profession. Its contemporary practice reflects both its history of caring and its influence by a range of global factors over time. The history of nursing is also the history of events that have occurred and continue to occur around the world. These include social evolution, the incorporation of multicultural perspectives, changing political regimes, wars, natural and human-made environmental impacts on health, shifts in the global economy, and the rise of new diseases, as well as the effects of increased efficiency of travel and advances in communication, genetics, and robotics, all of which have altered society's social systems. Nursing has been transformed by these and other changes that have influenced our health care system as a whole and the role of the nurse within it.

This book will help you understand the significance of the transformation in nursing and the profound influences these changes have had on our approach to nursing practice today. These changes range from the use of leeches to cure the ill to the use of technology and science in patient care, and also reflect the impact of shifts in the political and social landscape and their effect on nursing education.

In exploring how nursing has been shaped by broader historical and current events, this book showcases the role of nursing and its key place within the development of medicine from ancient and medieval times to the present. It reviews the role of religion in the responsibility of caring for the ill and illuminates how, even before modern scientific and medical advances, caregivers drew on specialized knowledge to deliver babies and tend to the sick. It delves into the unique role of the nurse in the care of the injured during wartime; traces the impact of key events, such as Florence Nightingale's effect on the care of soldiers during the Crimean War and nursing's role in subsequent wars on today's practice of nursing; and describes the future of health care and its direct influence on the nursing profession.

As you read each chapter, you will be introduced to global perspectives and key historical events that have had a profound impact on health care today. These are vital to understanding our role as nurses. In this way, we can apply new knowledge and perspectives, righting our course from paths previously thought to be effective for care that now are understood in a new light. Indeed, in attending to this history, we are reminded of the famous quote by George Santayana, "Those who cannot remember the past are condemned to repeat it" (*The Life of Reason*, 1905).

**Marilyn Klainberg, EdD, RN**
Professor and Department Chair
College of Nursing and Public Health
Adelphi University
Garden City, New York

# Preface

The history of the nursing profession used to be part and parcel of most nursing programs. However, myriad changes in health care, nursing, and technology have left little room to include this important content in nursing curricula. Today, many nursing programs gloss over this information because the curriculum is overburdened with content. However, most historians concur that learning about a profession's history provides its practitioners with a greater understanding and appreciation of the issues that inform their current and future practice and policies.

The history of the nursing profession is closely intertwined with that of health care, medicine, society, and public policy. Throughout the years, nurses have played pivotal roles in the health and welfare of populations across the life span and around the world. Recognizing the significance of the past on our current and future profession, the American Association for the History of Nursing advocates for the inclusion of nursing history in nursing curricula, and several nursing programs have developed resources about nursing's rich and diverse past.

There is a great need for a new book on the history of nursing, because many of the books on this topic were written more than 30 years ago. Of those available, few include the global perspective or devote more than one chapter to this subject in a large foundational textbook. *Fast Facts About the Nursing Profession* meets this need by helping nurses understand the important events and influential nurses that shaped nursing as a professional practice discipline. The book provides key information in an easy-to-read format, with "Fast Facts in a Nutshell" identifying key points throughout every chapter.

The book includes an interview with a nurse historian, Dr. Jean Whelan (conducted shortly before her death); a chapter on the relevance of nursing history by Dr. Brigid Lusk; and another chapter on pioneers in nursing and social activists by Dr. Donna M. Nickitas.

This book provides a brief historical overview of the origins of nursing and the profession. Each chapter highlights significant events around the world, the role of nurses, and the nursing profession in a particular era. The book begins in the pre-Nightingale era and includes the role of the nurse before formal training programs were developed. The significant and important relationship of nursing to medicine is also highlighted. The focus then moves on to Florence Nightingale and her significant contributions to nursing. Next, the focus shifts to the early 1900s and new developments in nursing, such as public health nursing, and the impact of both world wars. The chapters that follow provide a more in-depth account that focuses on the tremendous growth and professional development over the past 100 years. The final chapters look closely at nursing theorists and leaders, nursing education, nursing research, professional organizations, and the future of nursing.

**Deborah Dolan Hunt**

# Acknowledgments

Writing a book is indeed a labor of love, and although one often writes in isolation, there are countless individuals who support, contribute, review, critique, guide, or advise.

First and foremost, I must acknowledge Margaret Zuccarini for her unending support, advice, friendship, and frequently needed spelling lessons. I would also like to recognize the rest of the team at Springer Publishing for their dedication and support. I must say I am truly blessed to work in a profession that is replete with caring, compassionate, and professional nurses. I would like to recognize several who so generously contributed to this book:

- Dr. Brigid Lusk for her chapter, "The Relevance of Nursing History and Why It Matters Today"
- Dr. Donna M. Nickitas for her chapter, "Pioneers in Nursing Education and Social Activism: Lavinia Lloyd Dock, Isabel Hampton Robb, and Mary Adelaide Nutting"
- Dr. Jean Whelan (1949–2017) for her powerful and moving interview on the history of nursing and the important work of the American Association for the History of Nursing
- Dr. Marilyn Klainberg, a mentor and friend, who penned the Foreword for this book

This book has been strengthened considerably by these generous and expert contributions.

I must also acknowledge my family and friends who always support and encourage me. There are too many to list; however, I certainly hope they all know how much I love and admire them.

I must acknowledge my darling children who have taught me so much about life and who support, encourage, and inspire me every day to follow my dreams. A special shout-out to Caryl, a friend for life—our daily conversations are the best; Patricia, another lifelong friend, who lives far but is always near; my cousin Patty, who is more like a sister to me; and Therese, who is not only my friend but my very own "Dear Abby"!

I consider myself lucky to have such wonderful colleagues at the College of New Rochelle who have all taught me something unique about life, nursing, and education. A special shout-out to Dr. M. Dreher (dean) and Dr. D. Simons (associate dean) who always support and encourage me.

I would also like to acknowledge the following librarians: Arlene Shaner at the New York Academy of Medicine (NYAM), and Jennifer Ransom, Kathleen Mannino, Christine Blay, and Teresa Pivak (managing secretary) at the College of New Rochelle.

Last, but certainly never least, I must always recognize my special friend and mentor, Dr. Connie Vance, my teacher when I was in grad school, my mentor as a new nurse educator, and a friend for life.

# Introduction to the History of Nursing Through the Eyes of a Historian: An Interview With Dr. Jean Whelan

***Dr. Jean Whelan (1949–2017) was the president of the American Association for the History of Nursing (AAHN).***

**1. When did you first become interested in the history of nursing?**

When I was growing up, history and geography were my favorite subjects. During that era, there were three main career choices for women: teacher, nurse, or secretary. I always knew I wanted to be a nurse, and once I began my career, I quickly began to realize the importance of knowing the history of why things were the way they were.

I was inspired to delve into policy during the 1970s nursing shortage. I wondered why we had not been able to solve this problem. After a time spent as a clinical nurse, I went into nursing education, where I often emphasized the history of health care for my students, as I saw a natural link between nursing and history. Just as the first thing nurses do is obtain a history from their patients, it's critical that nurses understand the historical context of the health care delivery system and events taking place within it.

**2. Can you share some of those pivotal moments (or experiences)?**

The nursing shortage of the 1970s was a pivotal moment. I wanted to identify the reasons for the shortage and analyze it using a historical evidence-based methodology. One major observation I made was that while new graduate nurses made excellent salaries, their salaries did not increase with experience. Consequently, nurses' earnings ended up being very flat. I then began investigating why nurses' wages did not increase with experience. Questions I explored included: Why was compensation for nurses low in comparison to similarly skilled professions? Did the fact that nursing was a predominantly female profession make the difference? Was nursing undervalued because it was viewed as being a caring profession and care work is traditionally undervalued in our society?

**3. What do you believe are some of the most pivotal moments in our nursing history?**

I identify four main eras as pivotal to the progress of the profession. The first was during the 1890s to 1900, when there was tremendous growth in the number of nursing schools. From 1873 to 1890, there were only about 15 to 20 schools. This number increased to around 600 to 800 by the early 1900s. This growth, which was driven by the significant advances in scientific medicine requiring professional caregivers to carry out new and more advanced treatments, resulted in a very large number of graduate nurses who fanned out across the country to deliver professional care in homes and hospitals. As they did so, professional nursing began to be seen as essential to the delivery of modern medical care. This phenomenon appeared not just in the hospital system but also in the public health sector that increasingly was viewed as critical to societal well-being.

World War I was pivotal on an international level, with professional nurses being required to deliver care for massive numbers of sick and wounded soldiers. This was somewhat opposite to what had occurred during the Spanish–American War, when professional nurses were not accepted as a given. In World War I, nurses seized the moment and advanced not just bedside care, but also made tremendous strides in public health. Whether in the many hospitals set up as part of the war effort or in the public health field, nursing roles became more advanced. In many cases, nurses serving during the war carried out what we would consider advanced practice roles today.

World War II represented another pivotal moment for several reasons. I'll explain just one of them. Prior to this, private-duty nursing was the major occupational field for nursing. It was during the World War II era that nurses completed the transition to hospital employment. This represented a major change in the ways nurses worked in the conditions of their employment. Private-duty nurses worked as independent contractors responsible for generating their own income and making their own choices about when and where they would work. Employment as staff nurses tied nurses to more stable employment but resulted in a loss of independence in terms of determining their working conditions.

The final pivotal moment I'd identify is the postwar era when nurses began moving into more complex roles with the advent of intensive care units and the nurse practitioner programs in the 1960s. The rise of advanced practice nursing was pivotal not just for the profession but for the entire health care system.

**4. In your opinion, who has been the most influential leader in U.S. nursing—in the 20th century? In the 21st?**

It's hard to identify one individual leader. However, Lillian Wald is one of the most important nurses of all time. She founded the Henry Street Settlement (1915) and was also instrumental in formation of the NAACP (National Association for the Advancement of Colored People). She also helped to establish a significant nursing program affiliated with the Metropolitan Life Insurance Company in which nurses were sent out to visit sick subscribers of the company.

Janet Geister (1920s) was an early health systems research analyst who advanced several innovative ideas on how to distribute and employ nurses in a more efficient and logical manner.

Estelle Massey Osborne and Mabel Keaton Staupers led the National Association of Colored Graduate Nurses during the mid-20th century. Their efforts succeeded in integrating the nursing profession and promoting social justice.

Lucille Petry Leone directed the Cadet Nurse Corps, the first expansive federal aid to nursing education during World War II.

Katherine Densford was president of the American Nurses Association (ANA) from 1944 to 1948.

Anne Zimmerman was ANA president from 1976 to 1978.

Claire Fagin was former dean of the University of Pennsylvania's School of Nursing and the university's interim president. The first woman to lead an Ivy League school, Fagin was influential in setting policy regarding education and practice for the late 20th and early 21st centuries.

The 21st century is difficult to determine at this time as history is still being made; however, Linda Aikin's work has positively influenced the profession.

**5. What movement (or period) in nursing has been most influential in pushing the profession of nursing forward?**

The late 20th to early 21st centuries have been tremendously influential as nurses dealt with more complex issues and were "coming into their own," enabled to practice to the full extent of their education, skills, and scope of practice. Nurses, always core and essential to hospitals, seized opportunities to take advanced practice roles in new and innovative ways, resulting in a much more empowered profession.

**6. In what year did you become a member of the American Association for the History of Nursing (AAHN)?**

I became a member in 1994 and 1995 when I was completing my doctoral studies.

**7. You are currently the president of AAHN. What are some of the key initiatives your association has focused on in the past 5 years? Can you share some of the future goals?**

One of the most important key initiatives is the research grant program. Each year, two grants are awarded to doctoral students and one to a doctorally prepared scholar. The grant program awards a stipend allowing scholars to carry out cutting-edge research. A present and future goal of the AAHN is to raise sufficient money expanding the research endowment to allow additional grants to be awarded.

The AAHN's annual conference is excellent and offers an opportunity for mentoring and a venue for paper and poster presentations. The 2015 conference was held in Dublin, Ireland. In 2016, the conference took place in Chicago, and in 2017, it will be held in Tampa, Florida.

The AAHN is working diligently to increase its membership, which has been difficult. Membership fees are relatively low.

**8. Many nursing schools provide a very brief overview of our rich history. Do you know of any programs that require a course on the history of nursing?**

I am not aware of any nursing programs that require a course on the history of nursing. Schools of nursing currently have large numbers of required courses that often preclude adding more requirements. Some programs offer a history course as an elective.

**9. Do you believe a course in nursing history should be part of the core curriculum? Why?**

Nursing history should be part of the core curriculum, but it does not have to be a stand-alone course. History can and should be included content in all courses. One essential factor in threading history throughout the curriculum is that the school needs to have a faculty member who has a strong background in historical research and possesses a critical view of history and can blend nursing history into the curriculum with ease.

**10. Typically, history of nursing is part of a professional roles and "issues" course. Can you offer any recommendations on how to include this important content if it is not already included in one of the courses?**

Nursing history should be included in all courses and taught by someone familiar with the content. Strategies that can assist schools to include history in courses include using media such as instructional films that introduce students to historical concepts, inviting guest speakers to classes, and holding special lectures that highlight the latest historical research findings.

Students can participate in study groups where history and policy are combined to develop student-led seminars. One focus that often appeals to students and is highly relevant to their learning experiences is to have students investigate the history and treatment of a particular disease and how and why that treatment changed over time. A project such as that provides a student with a perspective that is different and more inclusive of learning about patient care.

**11. What advice would you offer a student or nurse who is interested in learning more about the history of nursing?**

I would advise students to join the AAHN and to seek out a mentor and make connections. For example, I am currently mentoring a BSN student who is completing her program and is doing her senior thesis on the role of nurses at Ellis Island. She reached out to me and we set up an agreeable arrangement with her adviser, which is working out wonderfully for both the student and me. Opportunities like that are easily available with just a little investigation for those interested. The AAHN is very willing to link students and nurses in general with historians who can mentor and discuss projects of a historical nature.

**12. Do you have any additional suggestions or comments?**

Currently, we are seeing a national resurgence in interest in history and in the history of nursing. If you think about recent events, such as the election of the first African American president and the nomination of the first female candidate of a major party for president, you see people thinking back on the past and placing into context the reasons why and how we got to this place as a nation. This is a good time for us to be thinking about why things are happening and where we are in nursing and health care. It helps us to make better plans for the future and places in perspective the role of nursing and nurses' role in the future.

# I

# The Origins of the Nursing Profession: Nursing Before Florence Nightingale

# 1

# The Relevance of Nursing History and Why It Matters Today

Brigid Lusk

Nursing history provides us the knowledge needed to understand our profession, learn from our past, and inform our patients and others about the significant role we play in health care. Throughout history, public opinion of nurses has shifted from one of disdain for the occupation to one of trust in the profession.

**In this chapter, you will learn:**

- How nursing history supports professional identity
- How awareness of history promotes critical thinking
- The history of patient care and of public opinion of nurses
- How diversity is represented throughout nursing history

A musty nursing textbook from 1942; a photograph of graduating nurses in long dresses and aprons, all wearing the same style of stiff, white cap; or a nurse's diary from a base hospital in France, written in 1917. What could these items have to do with you? Yes, they might be interesting—but can they help you practice as a nurse in today's high-tech health care world? I believe they can. This chapter is arranged to follow the key points of my argument:

- Nurses have a well-established history that supports professional identity and, therefore, retention in the profession.
- Nursing history is complex, with conflicting messages from society and from employers. Thus, appreciating our history requires critical thinking.
- Patients, silent in most social and professional histories, have a voice in the history of nursing. Hearing that voice, albeit from years past, enhances the practice of nursing.
- Understanding nursing history allows you, as a nurse, to inform the public about our history—rather than allowing the media or interested stakeholders to inform them.
- The history of nursing introduces students to the diversity of nursing practice, which, in turn, may open up previously unknown career opportunities.

**Fast Facts in a Nutshell**

"Nursing and history do sit on opposite sides of the science/arts divide. . . . Given this polarity, the point of nursing history for nursing practice has to be demonstrated rather than assumed" (Borsay, 2009, p. 17).

## HISTORY AND PROFESSIONAL IDENTITY

We can readily appreciate that a long professional history instills pride. Nursing has been a part of humanity's work, in all parts of the world, since the beginning of time. Long before Nightingale, long before the religious orders, people were caring for people who were injured or ill. It is part of being human. And these people practiced to the extent to which nursing and scientific knowledge were understood at that time. If their techniques seem strange to us today, it is because we practice at a later time with a different understanding of the human body's pathology. Even advanced practice registered nurses are not new. Nurses practiced anesthesia on the battlefields of the Civil War—more than 150 years ago (Keeling, 2007). In recorded history, midwives were the sole support of birthing women until giving birth became medicalized in the 18th century (Wertz & Wertz, 1989). Visiting nurses were the nurse practitioners for the poor in the 19th and early 20th centuries, and clinical nurse specialists evolved as in-hospital care became more critical.

One disturbing tendency Nelson and Gordon (2004) note is that nurses are adept at eliminating bothersome parts of their history and trying to start anew. This can include needlessly criticizing the skills of different types of nurses. The arguments go like this:

- Nurses in the early 20th century did little besides maintain cleanliness and comfort (Dingwall & Allen, 2001, as cited in Nelson & Gordon, 2004).
- Nurses with a baccalaureate degree (in the United States) are real nurses, unlike those with less education.
- Advanced practice registered nurses do not function as nurses compared with ordinary bedside nurses (Nelson & Gordon, 2004).

Thus, nurses have, in a vain effort to promote their standing, denigrated their broader and longer history. Nelson and Gordon (2004) have termed this the "rhetoric of rupture" and remind us that other professions, notably medicine, have not done this. Furthermore, by asserting that their fellow nurses have, purportedly, less knowledge and skills, the profession merely hurts its own image in the public's understanding of nursing. In addition, nurses' special knowledge of using herbs and fashioning poultices, for example, has been repudiated in favor of new skills (Nelson & Gordon, 2004). This self-immolating strategy of nurses devaluing their history bodes poorly for nursing today.

**Fast Facts in a Nutshell**

In 1900, the usual course of study for a medical doctor in the United States was 12 weeks of lectures that were then repeated; that is, the lectures were given twice. Nurses trained for 3 years (Lusk & Robertson, 2005).

## HISTORY AND CRITICAL THINKING

The history of nursing is not one-dimensional; it is complex in itself but must be factored within the contexts of time, place, gender, race, and innumerable other variables. Questionable treatments in which nurses participated, including lobotomies for the mentally ill, involuntary sterilizations, ultraradical surgeries for cancer, and aversion therapy for homosexuals, present opportunities for critical deliberation. Although controversial today, these historical case studies, because of the passage of time, can facilitate calm yet critical discussion.

Awareness and discussion of nursing's past promote analytical and effective thinking abilities among nurses, thus provoking this chapter's questioning of today's practice. For example, Tommy Dickinson's (2015) book, *"Curing Queers,"* concerning methods to "cure" homosexuality in the United Kingdom during the 1950s and 1960s, prompts one to ask the following question: What do we term an illness today that will have future nurses shaking their heads? History invites this type of questioning.

A bonus of this type of thinking is improved debating and writing skills. A complex argument requires mental organization. In turn, this promotes clear and persuasive arguments. All practitioners will be more effective if they have the skills to state their case clearly and write well. For nursing, this supports both patients and professional standing.

## HISTORY OF PATIENTS

The point of health care is to help an individual who is usually called a "patient." Patients are the most important players in any health care scenario, yet they are often silent. The history of nursing is inviolably bound to the history of patients with the advantage that nurses are not ill, not wearing a hospital gown, and not terrified of being in a strange place. Nurses can, thus, speak to the history of patients. As historian Anne Borsay (2009) notes, historical narratives of the nurse–patient relationship offer "flesh and blood examples to keep the recipients of health care in the frame" (p. 22).

Today, we are all bombarded with surveys. "How was our service?" "How was your stay?" "How easy was this survey to complete?" Annoying though these are, their point is to improve service and thus retain customers. Hearing the voices of patients enables nurses to provide better care. Lusk's (2010) account of a patient who had had a colostomy in 1951 can give some idea of what I mean. He had been discharged to a rehabilitation unit to learn how to manage his new colostomy.

> Had an awful time there at first. . . . Was irrigating lge. bowel with 10 cans a day. One nurse told me "we don't help people up here." Said I would have to do it myself. I didn't know where

> the bathroom was or what the set-up was. I didn't irrigate for three days, and it was awful. Then that nurse was "Off" and a nice little one was on. She took me up to the room, had a hook put up for me where I could reach it to put my own water in the can, she cut the tube off for me so that it would fit better, and everything went fine. (Lusk, 2010, p. 129)

It is worth noting that historians of medicine typically do not include the patient in their histories because the patient is not the primary point—it is the curative action itself, the surgery or the drug. The surgeon who performed the colostomy in the previous example might have written about the surgery and perhaps even about the man's immediate recovery, but would not have followed him through his stay, 24 hours a day, in the rehabilitation unit. Historians of nursing can reap these examples and share them. Nurses can benefit from these scenarios in their day-to-day practice of nursing.

## HISTORY AND PUBLIC OPINION OF NURSES

Many people have heard of Florence Nightingale, the acknowledged founder of modern nursing. She is almost universally revered. But what have people heard about the hundreds and thousands of women and men around the globe who have practiced as nurses?

Annie Holme (2015) reminds us that most people get their history from movies, fictional dramas, television, and museums. But the History Channel and even museums do not give a nuanced interpretation of nursing practice. Their history is simplified and sanitized and lacks critical awareness (Holme, 2015). Nursing history that the public does not get to see is so much richer. For a small example, think of nurses' uniforms. Old uniforms that we see are usually sparkling and fresh, possibly even newly made to duplicate the old style, perhaps for a museum or exhibition. In the Midwest Nursing History Research Center in Chicago, there are dozens of genuine old uniforms. Many of them are student nurses' uniforms from the 1880s and 1890s. These students nursed Chicago's poor in the Cook County Hospital. There are large semicircles of sweat stains under the arms, produced as nurses cared for patients in the blistering heat of a Chicago summer. All the windows would have been open; flies were a problem; there were scores of patients to care for. The aprons have many stains on them—from blood? From vomit? From dripping medicine bottles as the nurse poured out doses into the little glass measuring cups?

We need history to tell us about these nurses and, in turn, for us to tell the public. Holme (2015) writes of nurses in the United Kingdom today. Politicians, echoed by the media, are asserting that education has ruined nursing. In the past "golden age" of nursing, nurses were characterized as a "caring, compassionate workforce, lacking ambition in terms of occupational status and academic aspirations" (Holme, 2015, p. 635). This, Holme asserts, is not justified empirically or qualitatively but has lessened the public's trust in nursing. Caring and compassion are almost impossible to quantify, then or now, and a causative link between more education and less compassion is completely missing. But the impact of these imagined conjectures of the "golden age" of nursing might result in less education for nurses. It will certainly negatively affect the good that nurses can do.

**Fast Facts in a Nutshell**

The myth of the "golden age" of nursing has a long history. In 1929, the Michigan State Medical Society reported, "Pupil nurses today are younger and less considerate than formerly. This is shown in their noisiness . . . the mechanical performance of duties and their lessened humility when mistakes are made. . . . The committee believes that nurses are over-educated" (Lusk & Robertson, 2005, p. 101).

In the past, hours of patient care were critical for cooling patients sweating with fever, cleaning the pustules of patients with smallpox, and tending children paralyzed with polio. Perhaps these factors were judged as more caring. Today, factors such as greater patient acuity (because we know the safest place for sick people is usually their home) and computerized charting (because an electronic medical record ensures continuity of care) are key in nursing. History enhances patient care by contextualizing as well as recording the depth and breadth of nursing practice. History can ensure that employers, funding agencies, and the public understand the work of nursing.

## HISTORY AND DIVERSITY OF PRACTICE

The history of nursing provides new nurses some appreciation of the range of places to which nurses have traveled and the enormous variety of people for whom nurses have cared. Madsen (2008) stresses that history gives students an appreciation of the work of nursing in the community. But it gives more than that. History explores the national and international humanitarian work of nurses as they travel to disaster areas, including war zones and those of nature. History tells us about the early 20th-century midwives of the southern United States, and through that history, we enter the world of Jim Crow laws and racial segregation. Through history, we can explore the tenement houses of New York or Chicago and accompany the visiting nurses who cared for these immigrant and minority families at the turn of the past century.

One of my students illustrates this point perfectly. I was teaching an elective course in the history of nursing. One assignment was to find an interesting website related to the history of nursing and give a short presentation on it. My student, a senior who was graduating at the end of the semester, found the site of Mary Breckenridge and the Frontier Nursing Service (FNS) she founded in Kentucky back in 1925. My student was fascinated. She actually traveled to Kentucky during the upcoming spring break and visited the FNS, and her plan was to explore its work when she graduated. If it had not been for history, this student would never have known about the nurses on horseback.

### Fast Facts in a Nutshell

The first two U.S. military casualties of World War I, Edith Ayers and Helen Woods, were nurses. They were killed through friendly fire in May 1917, while onboard a ship traveling to France. During gunnery practice, portions of the brass cup of a shell boomeranged and killed the two nurses. Ayers and Woods were part of the U.S. Army Base Hospital 12 (Chicago Unit; Piemonte & Gurney, 1987, as cited in Gavin, 2006).

## SUMMARY

The relevance of the history of nursing to the practice of nursing can be found if one searches for it. Unlike the immediacy of pain or the urgency of a critical disease, the history of nurses can be silent. But it must not be. It is too important for our practice and our profession and our patients.

## References

Borsay, A. (2009). Nursing history: An irrelevance for practice? *Nursing History Review, 17*(1), 14–27.

Dickinson, T. (2015). *"Curing queers": Mental nurses and their patients, 1935–74*. Manchester, United Kingdom: Manchester University Press.

Gavin, L. (2006). *American women in World War I: They also served*. Boulder: University Press of Colorado.

Holme, A. (2015). Why history matters to nursing. *Nurse Education Today, 35*(5), 635–637.

Keeling, A. (2007). *Nursing and the privilege of prescription, 1893-2000*. Columbus: The Ohio State University Press.

Lusk, B. (2010). Nursing patients with cancer in the 1950s: New issues and old challenges. In P. D'Antonio & S. B. Lewenson (Eds.), *Nursing interventions through time: History as evidence* (pp. 123–138). New York, NY: Springer Publishing.

Lusk, B., & Robertson, J. F. (2005). US organized medicine's perspective of nursing: Review of the *Journal of the American Medical Association*, 1883–1935. In B. Mortimer & S. McGann (Eds.), *New directions in the history of nursing* (pp. 86–108). New York, NY: Routledge.

Madsen, W. (2008). Teaching history to nurses: Will this make me a better nurse? *Nurse Education Today, 28*(5), 524–529.

Nelson, S., & Gordon, S. (2004). The rhetoric of rupture: Nursing as a practice with a history? *Nursing Outlook, 52*(5), 255–261.

Wertz, R. W., & Wertz, D. C. (1989). *Lying-in: A history of childbirth in America*. New Haven, CT: Yale University Press.

# 2

# Nursing and Medicine in Ancient Times

The origins of nursing, medicine, and hospitals can be traced to ancient times, as early as 3000 BCE (Walsh, 1929). The history of nursing is so closely intertwined with medicine and health care that it is not possible to follow nursing's history without including the significant relationship and impact of medicine and the evolution of hospitals. The foundation of medicine as we know it today can be traced to Hippocrates, while nursing has evolved quite significantly from servant, to wet nurse, to handmaiden, to nurse-midwife, to the untrained nurse, and finally around the days of Florence Nightingale to the beginnings of the professionally trained nurse. It is posited that the role of the nurse during ancient times was most often fulfilled by servants, the poor, and at times family members.

**In this chapter, you will learn:**

- The origins of nursing, medicine, and ancient hospitals
- The roles of nurses and physicians between 3000 BCE and CE 1000
- The evolution of nursing during this period

## EARLY HISTORY OF NURSING

The earliest accounts of nursing date back more than 5,000 years to ancient Egypt, and in these and later accounts from Babylon, India, Greece, and Rome, nursing activities seem to have been aimed mainly at caring for the well-to-do. Two notable exceptions to the practice of neglecting the poor were documented. The first, in the Near East, was among Jews who subscribed to the Mosaic Code and had houses for the ailing; the second was among the Irish, who built a hospital in 300 BCE, which cared for both rich and poor (Walsh, 1929).

## ANCIENT EGYPTIANS

Ancient Egypt's physicians were influenced by their belief in the gods, who were thought to bestow on them the power to heal (Di Stefano, 1996; see Exhibit 2.1). Egypt had facilities known as "temple hospitals" (Walsh, 1929). The first physician on record, Imhotep, was a powerful minister and the personal physician to Zoser, a pharaoh who ruled during the Third Dynasty (during the 27th century BCE; Di Stefano, 1996, para. 6).

While ancient Egyptian physicians relied on spells and magic for healing and sought influence from the gods, evidence suggests that they also used herbs and plant extracts, including castor oil and opium, to treat a variety of conditions. The study of mummies has revealed that the Egyptians suffered from conditions such as rheumatoid arthritis and cirrhosis of the liver (Di Stefano, 1996).

Exhibit 2.1

### Influence of Ancient Mythology on Care of the Sick

- Egyptian mythology: Thoth was the "patron god of the physicians" and gave doctors the power to cure.
- Greek mythology: Hermes was the patron god of physicians.
- Egyptian and Roman mythology: Isis was known as the "goddess of healing" or earth mother goddess, and her influence was present in both Egyptian and Roman cultures (Di Stefano, 1996).
- Public institutions employed men to care for the ailing, while women ministered to the sick in their homes (Walsh, 1929).

In 1907, a study was undertaken along the banks of the Nile to explore cemeteries, examine bodies, and preserve ancient relics. Several important findings were made during the pathological examination of thousands of skeletons from various periods dating back to the predynastic era. They revealed that ancient Egyptians were afflicted with several diseases that are common today—renal calculi and gout were identified—however, there were no signs of syphilis or the skeletal changes associated with rickets, and tuberculosis was uncommon ("Ancient Egyptians," 1911/2011).

### Fast Facts in a Nutshell

"Ancient Egyptians" (1911/2011) relates that ancient Egyptian bodies were embalmed using the following process. The viscera were removed and the body pickled with a salt brine and then left out in the sun to dry. Once dry, the body was wrapped in a "mummy cloth," which helped preserve the body. Upon examination by modern scientists, different layers of the skin were recognized, renal tubules were present, and amino acids were noted in mummified tissue. The ancient Egyptians used advanced methods of embalming and mummification that led to the preservation of bodies for thousands of years.

## MEDICAL PRACTICES DESCRIBED IN THE BOOK OF EXODUS

According to Yee (2009), who used the texts of Exodus 1–2 from the Old Testament, medical practices among the ancient peoples of the Middle East were quite advanced. During the time of Moses (1393–1273 BCE), wet nurses, midwives, and slaves who were part of a marginalized group of citizens provided medical and nursing care (Yee, 2009). Renouard (1856) notes that hygiene was of tantamount importance during this period, and many animals were deemed impure. Among the writings contained in Leviticus is an account of the message that Moses received regarding childbearing. Cleanliness is described, in addition to the practice of circumcision for newborn males. There is also discussion of leprosy and how it should be treated: by priests who would then deem the patient unclean. The patient would be isolated so as not to spread the disease.

Some of the practices noted include the following:

- Midwives assisted in the birthing process.
- Midwives Shiphrah and Puah protected Hebrew babies against the pharaoh's decree of genocide.
- A wet nurse (*mêneqet*, which means "to suckle" in Hebrew) was selected by the father.

The *mêneqet* had to have the following qualifications: be aged 20 to 40 years, have given birth at least twice, have a healthy body, and have medium-sized breasts. Some *mêneqets* were paid, while others were slaves (Yee, 2009).

## BABYLONIANS

Historical records from Babylon describe the Code of Hammurabi, which provided legal guidelines for physicians who were paid for their services (Walsh, 1929). The laws contained in this code served two purposes: (a) outlining a fee schedule for surgical procedures and (b) formalizing what is considered to be the first known code of medical ethics (Forbes, 1935).

**Fast Facts in a Nutshell**

When medical services were provided, ancient Babylonian physicians could charge fees according to the patient's status or wealth. For example, a charge for a rich man could be five times as much as that for a slave (Walsh, 1929).

## ANCIENT GREEKS

During antiquity, the ancient Greeks developed the scientific foundations of medicine and philosophy, which guided their way of thinking (Kleisiaris, Sfakianakis, & Papathanasiou, 2014). In the Greek pantheon, Hermes was the god of medicine (see Exhibit 2.1). During the classical period (known as the "golden age" or "Age of Pericles"), a new paradigm was developed by Hippocrates (ca. 470–360 BCE), who is considered the "founder of Ancient Greek medicine" as well as medicine in general (Kleisiaris et al., 2014, p. 2). Hippocrates's approach focused on the natural treatment of a disease. Hippocratic medicine required the physician to:

- Study anatomy
- Practice holistically
- Focus on environmental and psychological factors, nutrition, and lifestyle
- Understand the need for a balance between the environment and the patient

Today, physicians still take the Hippocratic Oath when they earn their medical degrees. The oath requires the physician to practice with benevolence, human dignity, and integrity (Kleisiaris et al., 2014).

### *Highlights*

- Cnidus, the first known medical school, opened in Greece in 700 BCE.
- Medicine at this time focused on restoring a balance within the body through humoral medicine.
- Humoral medicine attempts to prevent and treat disease by restoring balance among four humors (blood, phlegm, and yellow and black bile) in the body (Alaeddini & Murty, 2014).

## ANCIENT INDUS PEOPLE

The ancient Indus peoples, like the Egyptians and Greeks, aspired to goodness for all humanity (Nutting & Dock, 1974). The highly developed Harrapan culture of the Indus valley (2300–1700 BCE) viewed water as the main purifying agent and source of life (Zysk, 1991). Dating back to the early Iron Age (about 1200–1000 BCE) is the *Atharvaveda,* a sacred text of Hinduism, which described the use of herbs for various ailments and the exorcism of demons (Sanujit, 2011). Hindus believed that there was an eternal maker and that in the beginning, people were free from sin and disease until they moved away from primal purity.

### Ayurveda

The traditional system of medicine known as Ayurveda (meaning "complete knowledge for long life") emerged around 1000 BCE, with

Table 2.1

**Ayurvedic Qualifications for Nurses and Physicians**

| Nurses | Physicians |
|---|---|
| ■ Purity of body and mind | ■ Purity of the mind and body |
| ■ Devotedness to the patient | ■ Cleverness |
| ■ Cleverness | ■ Large experience |
| ■ Knowledge of compounding and administering drugs | ■ Mastery of the scriptures |

*Source:* Nutting & Dock (1974).

the texts of Charaka (born ca. 600 BCE) and Sushruta (born ca. 600 BCE) being the most famous (Mukherjee & Wahile, 2006. The books of the *Ayur-Veda* are organized into eight parts that describe how to treat various diseases with medicine and surgery, including:

- Medical diseases
- Poisons and antidotes
- Demon possessions
- Children's diseases
- Genitourinary diseases
- Disease prevention through good hygiene practices

Historical records highlight the pivotal role that nurses played in ancient India. Both nurses and physicians were required to have specific qualifications (see Table 2.1).

## Buddhism

In a community established in India in the fifth century BCE, Buddhist monks served as healers mainly to fellow monks and used food and medicine in healing (Zysk, 1998). Nurses assisted in this care and, in order to be competent, had to provide medicine. The nurse is referred to as "he," which may mean that the nurse was male. The nurse was also required to clean the patient and remove mucus, urine, feces, and vomit. He was also expected to delight and gladden the sick by telling the patient a story from the Buddhist doctrine (Zysk, 1998, p. 42). These health practices and qualifications are very similar to current-day practice.

## ANCIENT CHINESE

Written accounts of ancient Chinese medicine date back more than 2,600 years before the Christian era. According to legend, P'an Ku, the first living person on Earth, lived to 18,000 years of age and then gave up his life for the benefit of the world. Wong and Lien-Teh (1973) point out that the creation of the myth of P'an Ku actually dates back to the fourth century CE and was brought to China by emissaries from Siam. During prehistoric times, healing was based on the supernatural, and there was limited knowledge of what actually caused diseases (Wong & Lien-Teh, 1973). The invention of medicine was attributed to the emperor Hoam-ti: "He is regarded as the author of a work entitled *Nuy'Kim*, which still serves as a guide to medical practice" (Renouard, 1856, p. 39). The book contains information about the pulse and the influence of hot and cold on various disorders.

### *Highlights*

- The Chinese practiced acupuncture with silver and gold needles, cupping, and hot and cold treatments, and they used various lotions and fomentations.
- Practitioners were knowledgeable about the cardiovascular and nervous systems.
- Extensive lists of pharmacopeia were developed.
- Practitioners did not perform surgical procedures.
- Ginseng root was one of the most important drugs used during this time (Renouard, 1856).

Wong and Lien-Teh (1973) argue that accounts of Chinese history can be dated reliably only to 722 BCE, which they describe as the start of "a glorious period in Chinese history" (p. 15). Two key doctrines evolved from the philosophies of Lao Tzu, Confucius, and Mencius. The first doctrine is the *yin* and *yang:* "Everything under the sun was supposed to originate from them" (Wong & Lien-Teh, 1973, p. 15). The *yin* and *yang* represent many opposite forces of nature—male and female, the sun and the moon, heaven and earth, positive and negative, and life and death. When it comes to health and illness, everything is classified as yin or yang according to its origins. "A disease is in *yang* when it is due to external causes and *yin* when it is due to internal causes" (Wong & Lien-Teh, 1973, p. 9). The second doctrine is the *five elements:* water, fire, earth, metal, and wood. According to this belief, the human frame is actually a mixture of these five elements, and if the balance of these is disrupted, the person will become ill. Five organ systems—heart, lungs, liver, spleen, and kidneys—relate to the five elements. In addition, in this system of medicine, four methods are used to diagnose diseases: observation, auscultation, interrogation, and palpation (Wong & Lien-Teh, 1973, p. 21). Notably, these methods of assessment are still used today.

**Fast Facts in a Nutshell**

Renouard (1856) asserts that the Chinese in particular have cultivated "Materia Medica and Pharmacology" (p. 43). Drugs were used to treat a plethora of diseases, with one of the most famous drugs being ginseng root, which was thought to cure a host of problems. Although the ancient Chinese were advanced in pharmacopeia, they did not perform surgical procedures.

## ANCIENT ROMANS

The Romans' practice of medicine was similar to that of the Greeks. Like the Greeks, they believed that the power to heal derived from the gods (in this case, Apollo and his son, Asclepius; see Exhibit 2.1). But their use of surgery and instrumentation was far more advanced. The Romans invented numerous surgical instruments, including the first instruments unique to the care of women, and established the surgical uses of forceps, scalpels, cautery, cross-bladed scissors, the surgical needle, the sound, and specula. Roman surgeons performed many procedures, including cesarean sections, cataract repair, and herniotomy. Surgical instrumentation was highly specialized, and more than 200 surgical instruments were found at Pompeii (Garrison, 1921). Roman physicians were also noted to treat malaria, gout, and different kinds of insanity.

## IRISH CELTS

The Celts migrated from Europe to Ireland around 1000 BCE. The Irish Celts were advanced in medicine and established many laws to guide medical practice. Physicians were trained by senior physicians, and "wise women" birthed babies. There was also a law of "sick maintenance" that provided for the needy and gave clear directions to the individuals who were caring for the sick. Of note, Princess Mach had the Broin Berg (House of Solrrow) hospital built in 300 BCE (Dolan, 1973).

**Fast Facts in a Nutshell**

Throughout ancient times, nursing is mentioned peripherally in some accounts and more formally in others that describe male and female attendants and midwives.

## SUMMARY

Historical records of medicine and nursing date back more than 5,000 years and demonstrate the significant advances that were made throughout the ancient period. It is fascinating to learn about many of the medical and nursing practices that began thousands of years ago and are still being used today.

### References

Alaeddini, A., & Murty, K. G. (2014). DSS (decision support system) for allocating appointment times to calling patients at a medical facility. In K. G. Murty (Ed.), *Case studies in operations research: Applications of optimal decision making* (pp. 83–109). New York, NY: Springer.

Ancient Egyptians and modern medicine. (1911/2011). *Journal of the American Medical Association, 305*(15), 1602. doi:10.1001/jama.2011.430

Di Stefano, V. (1996). The medicine of ancient Egypt: In Im-hotep's shadow. *Journal of the Australian Traditional-Medicine Society, 2*(1), 9–12.

Dolan, J. (1973). *Nursing in society: A historical perspective.* Philadelphia, PA: W. B. Saunders.

Forbes, R. (1935, September). A historical survey of medical ethics. *British Medical Journal, 2*(3897), 137–140.

Garrison, F. H. (1921). *An introduction to the history of medicine: With medical chronology, suggestions for study and bibliographic data.* Philadelphia, PA: W. B. Saunders.

Kleisiaris, C. F., Sfakianakis, C., & Papathanasiou, I. V. (2014). Health care practices in ancient Greece: The Hippocratic ideal. *Journal of Medical Ethics and History of Medicine, 7,* 6–10.

Mukherjee, P. K., & Wahile, A. (2006). Integrated approaches towards drug development from Ayurveda and other Indian system of medicines. *Journal of Ethnopharmacology, 103*(1), 25–35.

Nutting, M. A., & Dock, L. L. (1974). *A history of nursing* (Reprint ed.). Buffalo, NY: Heritage Press.

Renouard, P.-V. (1856). *History of medicine, from its origin to the nineteenth century, with an appendix, containing a philosophical and historical review of medicine to the present time.* Cincinnati, OH: Moore, Wilstach, Keys.

Sanujit. (2011, May 1). Religious developments in ancient India. In *Ancient History Encyclopedia*. Retrieved from http://www.ancient.eu/article/230/

Walsh, J. (1929). Date of Galen's birth. *Annals of Medical History, 1,* 378–382.

Wong, K. C., & Lien-Teh, W. (1973). *History of Chinese medicine: Being a chronicle of medical happenings in China from ancient times to the present period.* New York, NY: AMS Press.

Yee, G. A. (2009). "Take this child and suckle it for me": Wet nurses and resistance in ancient Israel. *Biblical Theology Bulletin, 39*(4), 180–189. doi:10.1177/0146107909343550

Zysk, K. G. (1998). *Asceticism and healing in ancient India: Medicine in the Buddhist monastery* (Corrected ed.). Delhi, India: Motilal Banarsidass.

# 3

# Nursing and Medicine: First Century CE to the Early Middle Ages

Beginning in the first century CE, medicine and nursing cycled between significant advances (e.g., the Salernitan Period) and less progressive periods (e.g., the Dark Ages). With the expansion of Christianity, there was a major shift in the care of the infirm (Walsh, 1929). "The Church made it one of the definite duties of churchmen, from the very beginning, to care for those in need, and especially those unable to care themselves, as during sickness" (Walsh, 1929, p. 1). The development of hospitals, and the need for doctors and attendants to serve them, continued to expand and paralleled the expansion of Christianity throughout the Middle Ages (Walsh, 1929). Although women were excluded from medical schools during this period, they did serve as midwives (Jones, 2009). Beginning in the first century of the Christian church, visiting nurses, "bearers of the lamp," provided care to those in need. These visiting nurses laid the foundation for what we consider community health nursing today (Dolan, 1973).

**In this chapter, you will learn:**

- What nursing and medicine were like during the early centuries CE
- How Christianity influenced nursing
- How nursing practice evolved in medieval times

## EVOLUTION OF THE NURSING PROFESSION

Beginning in ancient times, there are accounts of individuals who provided nursing care. For the most part, the nurses were unskilled and received no formal training. Indeed, many were poor and were provided minimal wages, and others were slaves who had no choice. However, there are also accounts of nurses who were expected to have certain qualifications. Furthermore, nurse midwives were in existence in ancient times and learned their skills by observing experienced midwives (Varney & Thompson, 2016).

## FIRST CENTURY CE

### Galen

The first century is remarkable for the influence of Galen (131–201 CE), considered one of the greatest Greek physicians after Hippocrates. He is also known as the founder of experimental physiology. He explained diseases using theory and treated patients with polypharmacy (Garrison, 1921). Galen published books on:

- Anatomy
- Physiology
- Pathology
- The pulse
- Medicine

He is credited with identifying inflammation and differentiating pneumonia and pleurisy, and "was the first to mention aneurysm" (Garrison, 1921, p. 104). He also identified the cranial nerves and the fact that arteries contain blood. Garrison (1921) points out that some of Galen's beliefs (e.g., on the physiology of the circulatory, nervous, and respiratory systems) were faulty, but these accounts were the only real knowledge on the workings of the human body for 17 centuries.

### The Romans

Interestingly, many accounts of Roman medicine are found in the writings of dramatists, poets, and secular writers (Garrison, 1921). Before the second century CE, the Romans used slaves and various individuals to perform many jobs associated with medicine; for example, medical slaves cared for the sick.

***Roles of Roman Slaves***

- Herb gatherer (*rhizotomi*)
- Salve dealers (*unguentarii*)
- Drug peddlers (*pharmacoplae*)
- Army surgeons (*medicic cohortis*)
- Body physicians to emperors (*archiatri*)
- Bath attendants (*iatrolipta*)
- Female healers (*sagae*)
- Midwives (*obstricae;* Garrison, 1921)

**Fast Facts in a Nutshell**

The Romans' attention to hygiene, as evidenced by well-ventilated houses, aqueducts, sewers, and drains, is of much greater consequence than their actual medical contributions, which are often regarded as being derived from the Greeks (Garrison, 1921).

## THE RISE OF ISLAM AND ARABIC MEDICINE

Arabic medicine emerged during the sixth century under the influence of Islam, founded in 570 CE by Mohammed. During this time, Arabic scholars were able to secure copies of various medical texts, for example, from Hippocrates, Galen, and Dioscorides. During the "Golden Age of Arabic Medicine" (Dolan, 1973, p. 61), the following contributions were made:

- Advancement of medical knowledge
- Compounding of drugs
- Description and treatment of disease

During the Mohammedan and Jewish periods, 732–1096 CE, the Mohammedan physicians received their medical knowledge from persecuted Christians (Garrison, 1921). Two notable physicians were:

- Ibn Sina (980–1036), a physician in chief to a hospital in Baghdad, who gave accounts of treating spinal deformities by forcible reduction and supported the use of wine for wound treatment

- Cordovan Avenzoar, a great Jewish physician who died in 1162; he described pericarditis, inflammation of the middle ear, and pharyngeal paralysis (Garrison, 1921)

## THE MEDIEVAL PERIOD (1096–1438)

The medieval period was a time of transition from ancient medicine that followed the fall of the Roman Empire. In the immediate aftermath, known as the Dark Ages, few medical advances took place. The most prevalent epidemic diseases were leprosy, epidemic chorea, and sweating sickness.

Neuburger classified medieval medicine into four periods:

- Monastic period (5th to 10th centuries), which focused on faith healing and the power of saints and holy relics
- Salernitan (11th to 12th centuries), which lifted medicine to a higher level
- Temporary enlightenment of the Arabist culture (13th century)
- Pre-Renaissance period (14th century; as cited in Garrison, 1921)

Monasticism was grounded in Christianity and other religions. During this time, individuals who wanted to lead good Christian lives could choose an occupation. The Benedictines, founded by St. Benedict (ca. 480–543), are a well-established monastic order that is still flourishing today. One of its most significant works was the care of the sick (Garrison, 1921).

**Fast Facts in a Nutshell**

St. Brigid (CE 452–523) "became a famous abbess in Ireland and a distinguished scholar, counselor, educator, and leader in the healing arts" (Dolan, 1973, p. 60).

### The Salernitan Period

The Salernitan period (in the 11th to 12th centuries) was associated with tremendous growth in medical knowledge and the development of the School of Salerno, which is credited as being the first independent medical school during this time. Students listened to lectures in the classroom and at the bedside. Methods of treatment included:

- Medications
- Psychotherapy
- Diet
- Bloodletting

There were also laws preventing the practice of medicine without careful examination. The program of study at the School of Salerno was quite rigorous and required 3 years of premedical study, 5 years of medicine and surgery, and 1 year of practice with an experienced practitioner. Quite notably during this time, women also studied at the School of Salerno (Dolan, 1973). From this period, medicine continued to expand and develop (Garrison, 1921; Renouard, 1856). "The chief glory of medieval medicine was undoubtedly in the organization of hospitals and sick nursing, which had its origin in the teachings of Christ" (Garrison, 1921, p. 168).

## Hospitals and Nursing During the Middle Ages

The religious crusades that took place from 1096 to 1291 resulted in the need for more hospitals and nurses to care for the injured. The development of military nursing orders resulted in large numbers of men entering the field of nursing. According to Carson (as cited in McSherry, 2006), during this time, hospitals were built to care for the pilgrims who were journeying to the Holy Land, such as the Knights Hospitallers of St. John for male patients. Hospitals were staffed by many workers responsible for cleanliness, linens, and meal preparation. There were also paid physicians and nurses in attendance. The *Deutscher Orden* (Teutonic Knights, founded in 1190) devoted their lives to defending holy places and caring for the poor and sick (Nutting & Dock, 1974).

Two famous hospitals were the Hôtel-Dieu (God's House) of Lyons and Paris. The hospitals were designed to care for the poor, the sick, the infirm, pilgrims, and children. The hospitals prospered for hundreds of years. Many of the nurses were "fallen women" who repented and wanted to lead a better life, while others were widows. At one point, they were called "*quasi-religieuses*" but, since the 1700s, have been known as "Sisters." Male nurses were originally called "servants" but, in later years, were known as "Brothers." Midwives practiced obstetrics and gynecology and often had a nursemaid in attendance during the birthing process. Physicians were consulted by midwives only when there was a difficult birth (Dolan, 1973; Nutting & Dock, 1974).

### Fatal Diseases

Three often-fatal diseases were:

- Leprosy
- Bubonic plague (the Black Death)
- Syphilis

As more people contracted communicable diseases, additional hospitals were necessary. According to Dolan (1973), the first hospital in England was in York in 936 CE, followed by St. Bartholomew's Hospital, which was built in 1123. "Later this hospital was made famous when it was used by Florence Nightingale as the center for clinical experience for her students" (p. 87).

### Notable Nurses and Nursing Orders

The following are a few notable nurses and/or nursing orders (Dolan, 1973; Nutting & Dock, 1974):

- St. Hildegarde (1098–1179)—considered a doctor and nurse
- Queen Elizabeth of Portugal (1271–1336)—created a hospital for foundlings and later joined the Poor Clares
- The Sisters of Charity, founded by St. Vincent DePaul—performed various acts of charity, such as nursing and teaching
- Three religious orders, founded by St. Francis of Assisi and St. Dominic—one for friars, one for nuns, and one for the laity
- *Deutscher Orden* (Germany)—nurses devoted their lives to defending holy places and to the care of the poor
- *Beguines* (Germany and Belgium)—a pious society devoted to nursing the rich and poor
- *Santo Spirito* (Rome, Italy)—primarily male nurses who developed hospitals and provided care to all

## SUMMARY

The period from the first to the 14th centuries was a time of significant advancements in medicine and, to a lesser degree, nursing. Indeed, the foundations of medicine, nursing, and health care were developed during this period. A greater understanding of the workings of the human body was realized, and formal medical training programs were developed. Most nursing care continued to be provided by unskilled men and women.

## References


Dolan, J. (1973). *Nursing in society: A historical perspective* (13th ed.). Philadelphia, PA: W. B. Saunders.

Garrison, F. H. (1921). *An introduction to the history of medicine: With medical chronology, suggestions for study and bibliographic data* (3rd ed.). Philadelphia, PA: W. B. Saunders.

Jones, C. (2009). Doctoring only for men? *HerStoria*, 15–18.

McSherry, W. (2006). *Making sense of spirituality in nursing and health care practice: An interactive approach* (2nd ed.). London, United Kingdom: Jessica Kingsley.

Nutting, M. A., & Dock, L. L. (1974). *A history of nursing* (Reprint ed.). Buffalo, NY: Heritage Press.

Renouard, P. V. (1856). *History of medicine, from its origin to the nineteenth century, with an appendix, containing a philosophical and historical review of medicine to the present time.* Cincinnati, OH: Moore, Wilstach, Keys.

Varney, H., & Thompson, J.B. (2016). *A history of midwifery in the United States: The midwife said* fear not. New York, NY: Springer Publishing.

Walsh, J. (1929). Date of Galen's birth. *Annals of Medical History, 1*, 378–382.

# 4

# Nursing From the Renaissance to the 18th Century

This chapter provides a brief overview of nursing and medicine from the Renaissance to the early 18th century. The influence of Christianity, medicine, and global issues on nursing is highlighted. Although the need for medical and nursing care increased in the 18th century, nursing continued to be viewed as a servile role, which was often relegated to the poor or indigent. The 18th century is often described as the "Dark Ages" of nursing due to squalid conditions of hospitals, poor care, and poor character of the nurses who worked in hospitals and the community (Funnell, Koutoukidis, & Lawrence, 2009).

**In this chapter, you will learn:**

- What nursing and medicine were like in the Renaissance
- The issues in nursing from the 1600s through the 1700s
- The relationship between medicine and nursing during the 18th century

## THE RENAISSANCE (LATE 14TH TO EARLY 17TH CENTURIES)

There was tremendous political, social, intellectual, and economic growth during the Renaissance. Less growth occurred in medical practice, which was replete with quackery, superstition, and herb doctoring. Furthermore, the practice of obstetrics was extremely unsafe until laws were enacted that required midwives to be employed to deliver babies and care for women's issues (Garrison, 1921). However, construction of hospitals in the 15th century expanded significantly, and there was a corresponding shift away from religious institutions as the providers of care (Garrison, 1921). During this period, plague and syphilis occurred in epidemic proportions.

Interestingly, in 1315, a professor named Mondini is credited with performing the first autopsies when he dissected the bodies of two women, which led to the publication of *Epitome of Anatomy.* The practice to some was barbaric, which led to a prohibition on anatomical dissection until the early 16th century. The physician Vesalius dissected corpses, and although his approach was highly controversial, his evident skill led to his appointment in 1537 as professor of surgery and anatomy at the University of Padua (Renouard, 1856). According to Renouard (1856), during the 16th century, anatomists were able to describe with exactness the easily accessible parts of the human body.

**Fast Facts in a Nutshell**

Nurses have been in existence since the beginning of time. Some civilizations had formal requirements for nurses, while others used slaves, the poor, or fallen women to serve as nurses. Christianity and the religious crusades had both a positive and negative impact on nursing.

## 17TH CENTURY

The 17th century was a time of significant medical advances throughout the world, including more precise anatomic illustrations, the discovery of circulation, the invention of the microscope, and advances in chemistry and physical science. Intravenous injections of drugs and blood transfusions were performed during this period. There were also notable advancements in obstetrics and the use of cesarean section (Garrison, 1921). A Ministry of Medical Affairs was created in Russia during the 17th century. Notably, Peter V. Postnikoff has been identified as the first native Russian physician; he studied in Italy and returned to Russia after graduating in 1694 (Garrison, 1921). Ireland also realized significant advances in medicine, with the formal training of physicians and implementation of practices based on the works of Galen. Many physicians served in the military. Many Irish physicians attended Charles University, a predominantly Catholic institution in Prague (Dillon, 2016). According to Wear (2000), medical practice in 17th-century England was provided by various practitioners. For example, charitable women or "white witches" were common providers in the villages, whereas top-end physicians provided care for the wealthy. Midwives, who usually were trained by other midwives, delivered babies; however, in the latter part of the 17th century, male midwives or surgeons provided care during difficult births.

## 18TH CENTURY

The 18th century was a time of great strife and unrest. Two wars—the American and French Revolutions—and catastrophic epidemics in England and America resulted in great loss of life (Dolan, 1973). The 17th to 19th centuries are considered one of the darkest periods for the nursing profession (Gabrielson, 1976). Furthermore, conditions were worse in big cities with poorly run hospitals and substandard care.

### Fast Facts in a Nutshell

Although both men and women served as untrained nurses in various capacities as in previous centuries, mothers provided most of the nursing care in the 18th century.

### Notable Nursing Contributions

The nurses who cared for the sick during the 18th century did not have formal training and, in comparison to their medical counterparts, were relatively stagnant educationally. However, they nurtured their patients and relied on creativity and ingenuity.

A few examples include (Dolan, 1973):

- Bed warmers to warm sheets
- Stone jugs filled with hot water to serve as heating pads
- Pewter cups for dry nursing
- Heating plates to make beef tea
- Herbal remedies

**Fast Facts in a Nutshell**

Many of these inventions and herbal remedies were based on folk healing and are still used today.

## Medical Advances

Several medical advances during the 18th century eventually affected the nursing profession, including Carl von Linné or Linnaeus's (1707–1778) attempts to classify diseases (although they later proved inaccurate; Mackenbach, 2004) and the birth of modern medical teaching in Great Britain with the teachings of William Cullen on chemistry, *materia medica*, and botany (University of Glasgow, 2015). With more doctors being prepared to practice, there was an increased need for nurses who learned through mentoring.

### *Highlights*

The following is just a brief overview of the myriad medical and scientific accomplishments during the 18th century (Dolan, 1973; Lyons, n.d.):

- William Cullen (1710–1790), professor at Glasgow and Edinburgh, developed the theory of "nervous energy."
- Leopold Auenbrugger's (1722–1809), *Inventum Novum* (1761) clearly outlined the procedure of percussing the chest (tapping with the fingers) to diagnose abnormalities of the thorax.
- Swiss Albrecht von Haller (1708–1777) described the current theory on the relationship between the cortex of the brain and the peripheral nervous system.
- Rene de Reaumur (1683–1757) invented a thermometer.
- Daniel Fahrenheit (1686–1736) made a glass thermometer in 1714.
- Herman Boerhave (1668–1738) was the first to use Fahrenheit's thermometer, which had to be placed against the body for 15 minutes.
- Stephen Hales (1677–1761) is credited with describing circulation and the capillary system and developing a manometer to measure blood pressure.
- Giovanni Battista Morgagni (1682–1771) identified renal tuberculosis, hepatic cirrhosis, pneumonic solidification of the lung, and syphilitic lesions of the brain.

## Discovery of Digitalis

The discovery of digitalis in 1785 by Dr. William Withering (1741–1799) is considered one of the most important medical discoveries during this century. Digitalis was used to treat dropsy (swelling of the limbs) and was developed based on a folk remedy (Lyons, n.d.). Interestingly, a nurse is credited with developing the folk remedy, which in turn led Withering to examine the herbal mixture. Through experimentation, Withering was able to extract digitalis, which was made from foxglove, and identify it as the drug for treating dropsy (Dolan, 1973).

### Fast Facts in a Nutshell

Many of today's practices, especially comfort measures, were developed by untrained nurses during the 18th century (Dolan, 1973).

## Epidemics in the 18th Century

Life-threatening epidemics occurred throughout the 18th century, due in part to a lack of education and unsanitary conditions. Diseases were also transmitted via ships by the individuals who were emigrating or trading (Rosenberg, 2008). These included:

**Early 1700s**

- Smallpox
- Diphtheria

**Late 1700s**

- Yellow fever
- Cholera (Rosenberg, 2008)

During the 1730s, an epidemic of diphtheria (referred to as "canker" or "throat distemper") affected thousands of children and young adults throughout New England; 5,000 died (Dolan, 1973; Rosenberg, 2008). Outbreaks of scarlet fever, another serious disease, were also common. Patients who survived but were weakened by one contagious disease sometimes succumbed to a second. In the late 18th century, 10% of the population in Philadelphia died due to an epidemic of yellow fever. Because there was such a shortage of nurses, the Free African American Society recruited African American nurses to care for those afflicted (Foster, Jenkins, & Toogood, 1993).

### Cowpox, Smallpox, and Inoculation, or Variolation

People living in Europe, Asia, and Africa experienced smallpox and cowpox epidemics throughout history. Various methods of treating the disease were developed, such as the Turkish method of scratching infected pus into the skin, which was introduced in Europe by Lady Mary Wortley Montagu (1689–1762). However, although this method had some positive effects, there were still many outbreaks (Riedel, 2005).

Two approaches to prevent smallpox became more widespread in the 18th century:

- Arm-to-arm rubbing—material dipped into the pus of an infected person was placed on a small incision of a healthy person.
- *Variolae vaccinae* (cowpox)—Edward Jenner pioneered vaccination for smallpox when he (correctly) deduced that infecting a healthy person with cowpox (a related but less serious disease) would confer immunity to smallpox (Riedel, 2005).

**Fast Facts in a Nutshell**

Smallpox has been virtually eradicated; however, in recent years, vaccination compliance has decreased, and recently there have been outbreaks of diseases such as the mumps and measles.

## SUMMARY

The medical and nursing professions from the Renaissance through the 18th century were greatly influenced by Christianity, with many advances after the Renaissance and a time of stagnation during the 18th century. It was also a time when fatal plagues and diseases occurred throughout the world. Interestingly, the development of vaccinations and medications such as digitalis can be traced back to the 18th century.

### Further Reading

Nutting, M. A., & Dock, L. L. (1974). *A history of nursing* (Reprint ed.). Buffalo, NY: Heritage Press.

## References


Dillon, C. (2016). Medical practice and Gaelic Ireland. In J. Kelly & F. Clark (Eds.), *Ireland and medicine in the seventeenth and eighteenth centuries* (pp. 39–52). London, United Kingdom: Routledge.

Dolan, J. (1973). *Nursing in society: A historical perspective* (13th ed.). Philadelphia, PA: W. B. Saunders.

Foster, K. R., Jenkins, M. F., & Toogood, A. C. (1993). Introduction to the 1993 edition. In J. H. Powell, *Bring out your dead: The great plague of yellow fever in Philadelphia in 1793* (Reprint ed., pp. ix–xvi). In J. E. Lynaugh (Series Ed.), Studies in Health, Illness, and Caregiving. Philadelphia: University of Pennsylvania Press.

Funnell, R., Koutoukidis, G., & Lawrence, K. (2009). *Tabbner's nursing care: Theory and practice* (3rd ed.). Melbourne, Australia: Elsevier.

Gabrielson, R. C. (1976). Two centuries of advancement: From untrained servant to skilled practitioner. *Journal of Advanced Nursing, 1*(4), 265–272. doi:10.1111/j.1365-2648.1976.tb00965.x

Garrison, F. H. (1921). *An introduction to the history of medicine: With medical chronology, suggestions for study and bibliographic data (3rd ed.).* Philadelphia, PA: W. B. Saunders.

Lyons, A. S. (n.d.). *Medical history—the eighteenth century.* Retrieved from http://www.healthguidance.org/entry/6351/1/Medical-History—The-Eighteenth-Century.html

Mackenbach, J. P. (2004). Carl von Linné, Thomas McKeown, and the inadequacy of disease classifications. *European Journal of Public Health, 14*(3), 225.

Renouard, P. V. (1856). *History of medicine, from its origin to the nineteenth century, with an appendix, containing a philosophical and historical review of medicine to the present time.* Cincinnati, OH: Moore, Wilstach, Keys.

Riedel, S. (2005, January). Edward Jenner and the history of smallpox and vaccination. *Baylor University Medical Center Proceedings, 8*(1), 21–25.

Rosenberg, C. E. (2008). Siting epidemic disease: 3 centuries of American history. *Journal of Infectious Diseases, 197*(S1), S4–S6.

University of Glasgow. (2015). A significant medical history: 18th century. Retrieved from http://www.gla.ac.uk/schools/medicine/aboutus/history/18thcentury

Wear, A. (2000). *Knowledge & practice in English medicine, 1550–1680.* London, United Kingdom: Cambridge University Press.

# 5

# Nursing Around the Globe in the 18th Century

This chapter highlights issues in nursing and medicine around the globe during the 18th century. Many countries faced similar hardships during this period, and the nursing profession was experiencing its darkest time in history. Nevertheless, devoted men and woman ministered to the infirm in homes, in hospitals, and even on the battlefield.

**In this chapter, you will learn:**

- The relationship between war and the care of the injured
- How conditions present in many hospitals affected the ill and injured
- Unique nursing roles and beliefs around the world

## COLONIAL-ERA NURSING IN AMERICA

During the 1700s, most care of the infirm was provided by family members in their own homes. However, many individuals were either too poor or too sick to care for themselves or their families. This led to the opening of an almshouse in 1732 in Philadelphia (Blaisdell, 1992). Because so many individuals in this setting also had serious illnesses, a section was created to care for them. Interestingly, Philadelphia General Hospital started out as an almshouse. A prevailing belief held that illness was a punishment from God; in fact, many of these primitive hospitals were likened to penitentiaries (Gabrielson, 1976).

The following hospitals were founded before the Revolutionary War:

- Bellevue Almshouse and New York Hospital, in New York City
- Blockley Almshouse (later Philadelphia General Hospital) and Pennsylvania Hospital, in Philadelphia
- A hospital for the insane, in Williamsburg, Virginia

In 1751, Pennsylvania Hospital opened as a private facility. Benjamin Franklin (1706–1790), one of the hospital founders, recognized the important role of nurses and posited that high-quality nursing care was vital in the restoration of health (Franklin, 1754).

### Fast Facts in a Nutshell

Stephen Girard, a wealthy French-born banker, won the hearts of citizens of his adopted city of Philadelphia for his courageous and compassionate nursing of the victims of the 1793 yellow fever epidemic (Girard, 1832).

## Nursing During the Revolutionary War

The Revolutionary War took place from 1775 to 1783, with more than 25,000 men losing their lives and countless others being injured (Peckham, 1958). During the war, many women took on roles that traditionally were filled by men who were now serving their country. Nursing was one of these roles; many were recruited and at times coerced and threatened to become nurses. These women had no choice, as they desperately needed the rations and the meager salary that was paid by the Continental Army (Danyluk, 1997). The list of duties outlined in Exhibit 5.1 highlights the menial, yet important, tasks for which many nurses were responsible during the Revolutionary War.

### *Highlights*

- General George Washington ordered many women to serve as nurses to the soldiers.
- Many wives followed their husbands so that they could nurse them back to health when they were injured.

Exhibit 5.1

**Nursing in the Revolutionary War**

The "Rules and Directions for the better regulation of the military Hospital of the United States" outlined the following nursing duties:

- Bathe new patients and comb hair daily
- Empty chamber pots
- Change linens
- Sweep the floors
- Sprinkle wards with vinegar, which was used as a disinfectant
- Seek permission to be absent and remain clean and sober (Danyluk, 1997)

- In 1775, a congressional resolution deemed that there should be one nurse for every 10 patients in the army hospitals.
- The nurses were paid $2 per month, which eventually was increased to $8 per month in 1777 (Danyluk, 1997).

**Fast Facts in a Nutshell**

At the Battle of Monmouth, Mary Hays, wife of an artillery man, brought water to clean the cannon, and when her husband collapsed, she assisted in firing it (Danyluk, 1997).

## CANADIAN NURSING AND THE FRENCH COLONIES

Canadian nursing traces its roots back to Marie Rollet Hébert, who assisted her husband, Louis Hébert, a surgeon-apothecary, in caring for the sick (Bennett, 2014). Nursing in much of French Canada was provided under the auspices of religious organizations. Among the groups providing care were the Sisters (Augustinians) of the Hôtel-Dieu, who cared for patients during several epidemics as well as the French and Indian War (Dolan, 1973; see Exhibit 5.2).

The practice of outreach nursing or "street nursing" in Canada can be traced back to the 1700s. Founded by Marie-Marguerite d'Youville, the Grey Nuns (also known as the Sisters of Charity) cared for the poor. In 1737, d'Youville, who was a young widow, began taking impoverished people into her home (Hardill, 2007). The order grew,

Exhibit 5.2

**Timeline of French Canadian Nursing: The Sisters (Augustinians) of the Hôtel-Dieu**

**1703**—Ministered to the infirm during a severe smallpox epidemic (2,000 lives lost)
**1710**—Cared for patients during the yellow fever epidemic
**1740**—Ministered to the plague patients who were brought in by ship
**1759**—Ordered to work at the General Hospital of Montreal and later to care for the soldiers during the French and Indian War (Dolan, 1973)

and by 1750, d'Youville and her colleagues had renovated the ruined General Hospital of Montreal and opened it as a home to all. Word among the destitute was "Go to the Grey Nuns; they never refuse" (Miller, n.d., para. 3).

**Fast Facts in a Nutshell**

The government attempted to restrain d'Youville's generosity (Miller, n.d.).

## ENGLAND

Nursing and health care in 18th-century England were similar to nursing in America. During the 18th century, nursing was part of women's role, along with housekeeping and raising children, and nurses grew herbs for healing and cooking (Marshall, 1983). There were two royal hospitals and several voluntary hospitals. Nursing was one of the most common female professions in London. The role of the nurse included:

- Sick nursing of adults
- Wet nursing of infants
- Dry nursing of children (London Lives, 2010)

According to London Lives (2010), there were nurses who were uncaring and ineffective, and some were drunkards. For example:

- Eleanor Gilmore was charged with neglectful care and murder but was found not guilty in 1718.

- Elizabeth Brownrigg was convicted of murdering a parish nurse apprentice named Mary Clifford in 1766.

## Fast Facts in a Nutshell

The Gin Act was passed in 1751 in an effort to alleviate the "gin epidemic" that occurred from 1720 to 1751 (Warner, Her, Gmel, & Rehm, 2001).

## NURSING CARE IN OTHER COUNTRIES

### Ireland

During the 18th century, most of the medical and nursing care throughout Ireland was administered in the home. During the 17th and 18th centuries, most Irish physicians were trained abroad, and unfortunately, many continued to practice outside of Ireland (Kelly & Clark, 2010). Thus, there were not enough physicians in Ireland, and very few patients used hospitals. Women assumed responsibility for providing medical and nursing care to their families. Although there was no formal training, there was experiential training and the use of "receipt books" (Kelly & Clark, 2010, p. 11) to record the various remedies that would be used when a person fell ill. These receipt books, which contained many herbal remedies, were passed down from one generation to the next and provided the foundation for nursing care prior to formalized training programs.

### France

Medicine and nursing in 18th-century France were similar to other parts of Europe and the United States. However, there were some unique differences. For example, there was a debate about the smallpox inoculation during the epidemic because the French were very apprehensive about the efficacy and safety of the inoculations. In an effort to improve the compliance rate, the statistical assessment of risk emerged during the 18th century, and in 1760, Daniel Bernoulli, a philosopher, offered a mathematical assessment of risk, which was 1 in 200 per inoculation. However, this did not convince the French that there was a greater risk in not being inoculated, and the medical community posited that the decision should be a familial one and not a government mandate (Lipkowitz, 2003). Another unique development in French nursing was the French Revolution, which took place in 1789 (Palmer, 2016) and led to an increased need for nursing and medical care.

### *Highlights*

- Hôtel-Dieu hospital in Paris was created and is still in existence today.
- Under the rule of Louis XIV, health care was provided to beggars, vagabonds, and the poor.
- The Paris Parliament headed the Paris general hospital and employed both secular and religious staff, who were often very knowledgeable apothecaries.
- Apothecaries opened small dispensaries, which resulted in improved health of the French (Diebolt, 2013).

## Germany

Literature on nursing in Germany and the surrounding countries during the 18th century is sparse. The Protestant Reformation resulted in the seizing of many monasteries and the hospitals that were housed in them (Bagwell, 2013; Yerby, 1967). This, along with the movement of people from rural area into towns, increased the role of government in providing health care to Germans (Yerby, 1967). This could have contributed to the decline of nursing nuns and the stagnation of nursing during the 18th century.

**Fast Facts in a Nutshell**

Homeopathy can be traced back to the 1700s, when Samuel Hahnemann developed a system whereby diseases were treated with drugs that resembled the effects of the disease, with the caveat being that minute amounts were administered (Teixeira, 2014).

## China

Medicine and health care in China were greatly influenced by the Buddhists and Taoists. The Buddhists believed that people became ill because they were being punished for some type of sin. In contrast, the Taoists believed that people became ill due to a spell or wrath of a deity. Because of these philosophical beliefs, there are few references to nursing because one could not interfere with divine plans, although wives and mothers did provide informal care in the home (Gage, 1919).

### India

Public health care in India in the 18th century was seriously lacking, with high mortality rates due to diseases such as plague, cholera, tuberculosis, smallpox, and malaria. India was under British rule and medical services were established, but they were primarily for the British soldiers, laborers, and civil servants (Kamalam, 2011).

### Africa and Its Influence on the United States

Care of the sick in Africa was based on folk healing and herbal medicine, as practiced by healers in the villages. Through the slave trade, these practices were spread to Europe and America. Healers among enslaved African peoples used native roots to treat fevers, especially when traveling on cargo ships, and amulets (necklaces with wild licorice seeds) for protection (Fett, 2002).

## CHRISTIANITY, CATHOLICISM, AND NURSING

It is a well-known fact that in the 18th century, most of the care of the sick and the indigent was provided by the Sisters in the various religious orders, which were grounded in the teachings of Christianity (Violette, 2005). According to Violette (2005), more than 50 religious orders were instrumental in the development of the Catholic hospital network in Canada.

#### *Highlights*

- Grey Nuns of Montreal—noted for their apothecary knowledge
- Sister Saint-Martin (1770–1832)—noted apothecary who performed surgery and served on the community planning board (Violette, 2005)
- Augustinian nuns—established hospitals, visiting nurse services, orphanages, and schools throughout Canada (Jamieson & Sewall, 1954; Nutting & Dock, 1974)

## SUMMARY

The 18th century was known as a dark period due to a lack of formal nursing training and many unskilled nurses who were actually unsavory characters. It is important to note that there were also some exemplary nurses, such as those of the various religious orders. During this period, much of the nursing care was provided by mothers and wives in the home, community, and even on the battlefield, especially in the Revolutionary War.

### References


Bagwell, C. E. (2013). Nosokomia to sacred infirmary: Legacy of the Knights Hospitaller and Chimbarazo Hospital in the evolution of hospitals from medieval to modern. *Journal of the American College of Surgeons, 216*(4), e35–e42.

Bennett, E. M. G. (2014, November). Rollet, Marie. In *Dictionary of Canadian biography* (Vol. 1). Retrieved from http://www.biographi.ca/en/bio/rollet_marie_1E.html

Blaisdell, F. W. (1992). 1991 A.A.S.T. presidential address: The pre-Medicare role of city/county hospitals in education and health care. *The Journal of Trauma, 32*(2), 217–228.

Danyluk, K. (1997). Women and the Revolutionary War. *Colonial Williamsburg Interpreter,* 8–13. Retrieved from http://www.history.org/history/teaching/enewsletter/volume7/nov08/women_revarmy.cfm

Diebolt, E. (2013). Prémices de la profession infirmière: De la complémentarité entre soignantes laïques et religieuses hospitalières XVIIe—XVIIIe siècle en France [The beginnings of the nursing profession: The complementary relationship between secular caregivers and hospital nuns in France in the 17th and 18th centuries]. *Recherche en Soins Infirmiers, 113,* 6–18.

Dolan, J. (1973). *Nursing in society: A historical perspective.* Philadelphia, PA: W. B. Saunders.

Fett, S. M. (2002). *Working cures: Healing, health, and power on Southern slave plantations.* Chapel Hill: University of North Carolina Press.

Franklin, B. (1754). *Some account of the Pennsylvania Hospital, from its first rise, to the beginning of the fifth month, called May, 1754.* Philadelphia, PA: Author & D. Hall.

Gabrielson, R. C. (1976). Two centuries of advancement: From untrained servant to skilled practitioner. *Journal of Advanced Nursing, 1*(4), 265–272. doi:10.1111/j.1365-2648.1976.tb00965.x

Gage, N. D. (1919). Stages of nursing in China. *American Journal of Nursing, 20*(2), 115–121. doi:10.2307/3405591

Girard, S. (1832). *Biography of Stephen Girard, with his will affixed; Comprising an account of his private life, habits, genius, and manners; Together with a detailed history of his banking and financial operations for the last twenty years* (2nd ed.). Philadelphia, PA: Thomas L. Bonsal.

Hardill, K. (2007). From the grey nuns to the streets: A critical history of outreach nursing in Canada. *Public Health Nursing, 24*(1), 91–97. doi:10.1111/j.1525-1446.2006.00612.x

Jamieson, E. M., & Sewall, M. F. (1954). *Trends in nursing history.* Philadelphia, PA: W. B. Saunders.

Kamalam, S. (2011). *Essentials of community health nursing practice* (2nd ed. rev.). New Delhi, India: Jaypee Brothers.

Kelly, J., & Clark, F. (Eds.). (2010). *History of medicine in context: Ireland and medicine in the seventeenth and eighteenth centuries.* Farnham, United Kingdom: Ashgate.

Lipkowitz, E. (2003). The physicians' dilemma in the 18th-century French smallpox debate. *Journal of the American Medical Association, 290*(17), 2329–2330. doi:10.1001/jama.290.17.2329

London Lives. (2010). *Parish nurses.* Retrieved from http://www.londonlives.org/static/ParishNurses.jsp

Marshall, R. K. (1983). *Nursing Mirror* history of nursing: Scottish hospitals in the 18th century. *Nursing Mirror, 156*(8), i–viii.

Miller, D. (n.d.). *Saint Marguerite d'Youville: Saint of the day for June 15.* Retrieved from https://www.franciscanmedia.org/saint-marguerite-d-youville

Nutting, M. A., & Dock, L. L. (1974). *A history of nursing* (Reprint ed.). Buffalo, NY: Heritage Press.

Palmer, R. R. (2016). *The world of the French Revolution.* London, United Kingdom: Routledge.

Peckham, H. H. (1958). *The war for independence: A military history.* Chicago, IL: University of Chicago Press.

Rosenberg, C. (2008). Siting epidemic disease: 3 centuries of American history. *Journal of Infectious Diseases, 197*(S1), S4–S6.

Teixeira, M. Z. (2014). "Paradoxical pharmacology": Therapeutic strategy used by the "homeopathic pharmacology" for more than two centuries. *International Journal of High Dilution Research, 13*(48), 207–226.

Violette, B. (2005). Healing the body and saving the soul: Nursing Sisters and the first Catholic hospitals in Quebec (1639–1880). In C. Bates, D. Dodd, & N. Rousseau (Eds.), *On all frontiers: Four centuries of Canadian nursing* (pp. 57–72). Ottawa, ON, Canada: University of Ottawa Press.

Warner, J., Her, M., Gmel, G., & Rehm, J. (2001). Can legislation prevent debauchery? Mother gin and public health in 18th-century England. *American Journal of Public Health, 91*(3), 375–384.

Yerby, A. S. (1967, March/April). Health departments, hospitals and health services. *Medical Care, 5*(2), 70–74.

# 6

# 19th-Century Nursing in the Pre-Nightingale Era and Beyond

The foundations of nursing as it exists today were laid during the early 1800s. Several factors played a part in the growth and expansion of nursing as a profession, and the Crimean War in Europe and the Civil War in America had a profound effect. The role of nurses in the early part of the 19th century was fairly similar to that in the 18th century; however, by the latter part of the century, conditions were vastly improved. Training programs were established, and Florence Nightingale had a major influence on health care, nursing, and nursing education. Nightingale's influence was so pervasive that her accomplishments are set off separately in another chapter. Refer to Chapter 7 for discussion of her work and significant contributions to the nursing profession.

**In this chapter, you will learn:**

- What nursing in the 19th century was like
- Who the influential nurses were during this period
- How nursing and medicine were influenced by the Civil War
- How the medical model influenced nurse-training programs
- The initial training programs in nursing

## NURSING IN THE EARLY 19TH CENTURY

Nursing in the early 19th century was fairly similar to the previous century, with untrained nurses working in hospitals and wives and mothers providing care in the home. In London, most of the nurses were actually domestic workers who were recruited to work in hospitals, where they performed similar duties (Wright, 1999). American society in the 1800s was influenced by urbanization, industrialization, and the Civil War. There were also several medical advances; these most often originated in Europe.

For example:

- Chloroform was used for pain relief.
- Morbidity and mortality were reduced by decreasing infections with the use of antisepsis.
- Hospitals became safer and more hygienic.
- Family units became smaller and more people worked out of the home, so the ill had to be treated in hospitals (Kalisch & Kalisch, 2004; Wawersik, 1997).

Nurse-training programs were developed to meet the demands for competent nurses for private duty and hospital work (see Exhibit 6.1).

Exhibit 6.1

### Timeline of Early Nurse-Training Programs

**1798**—Valentine Seaman, a New York physician, organized an early course of lectures for nurses who care for maternity patients.

**1828**—Nurse-Midwifery Program in Philadelphia established; Dr. Joseph Warrington trained and awarded nurse-midwives a Certificate of Approbation.

**1860**—Florence Nightingale established the St. Thomas Hospital Nursing School, which became the model for many nursing schools.

**1869**—Women's Hospital of Philadelphia offered a 6-month nurse-training course, which graduated its first class in 1869.

**1872**—The New England Hospital for Women and Children founded the first nursing school that awarded a nursing diploma.

**1873**—The New York Training School at Bellevue Hospital, the Connecticut Training School at the State Hospital, and the Boston Training School at Massachusetts General Hospital developed "Nightingale schools" based on the principles set forth by Florence Nightingale (Condon, 2001; Kalisch & Kalisch, 2004)

**Fast Facts in a Nutshell**

Linda Richards, who graduated in 1873, was the first nurse to receive a nursing diploma, and Mary Mahoney, who graduated in 1879, was the first American Black nurse to graduate from the New England Hospital for Women and Children's Nursing School (Condon, 2001).

## NOTABLE NURSES OF THE 19TH CENTURY

There were many influential nurses during the 19th century, and the following list highlights their many contributions. It is important to note that this is not an all-inclusive list.

**Dorothea Dix (1802–1887)**

- Superintendent of army nurses during the Civil War
- Advocate for the mentally ill (Sitzman, 2010)

**Mary Seacole (1805–1881)**

- Jamaican nurse who cared for patients during the Crimean War
- Delivered medicine and food
- Learned about herbal medicines from her mother, who was Jamaican (Ellis, 2009; Robinson, 2004)

**Mary Todd Lincoln (1818–1882)**

- Married to President Lincoln
- Volunteer nurse who served in the Civil War (Miller, 2006)

**Walt Whitman (1819–1892)**

- Volunteer nurse during the Civil War
- Famous poet
- Wrote *Memoranda During the War,* which chronicled the Civil War (Sitzman, 2010)

**Florence Nightingale (1820–1910)**

- Founder of modern-day nursing
- Served in Crimean War—influential nurse known for hand hygiene and cleanliness on wards
- Penned *Notes on Nursing,* which focused on hygiene, diet, holistic care, and nursing theories (Nightingale, 1860)
- Founder of Nightingale Nursing School, which most schools model today

**Clara Barton (1821–1912)**

- Served in the Civil War
- Founded the American Red Cross in 1881 (Kalisch & Kalisch, 2004)

**Linda Richards (1841–1930)**

- First American-trained nurse
- Graduated from the New England Hospital for Women and Children's School of Nursing in 1873
- Established nursing schools in the United States and Japan
- Developed a method of charting and recordkeeping for hospitalized patients (Detar, 2009)

**Mary Mahoney (1845–1926)**

- First African American professional nurse
- Graduated from "one of the first accelerated nurse training programs" (Sitzman, 2010, p. 40)
- Cofounded the National Association of Colored Graduate Nurses (merged with the American Nursing Association in 1951; Sitzman, 2010)

**Jane Elizabeth Hitchcock (1863–1939)**

- Public health nurse
- Advocated for the integration of public health nursing theory and clinical experiences into training programs (Hawkins & Watson, 2003)

**Lillian Wald (1867–1940)**

- Founder of American Community Nursing (Sitzman, 2010)
- Advocate of equal care for the poor and immigrants (Fee & Bu, 2010)

## NURSE MATRONS IN 19TH-CENTURY ENGLAND

Nursing in the early part of the 19th century left much to be desired. Nursing was considered a lowly profession, and the nurses were untrained and performed menial tasks. For example:

- Making beds
- Bathing patients
- Cleaning and emptying bedpans
- Making poultices (Helmstadter, 2008)

The nurses were paid a small wage, were expected to work 16-hour shifts, and usually lived in the attics or cellars of the hospitals where they worked. The hospitals were run by matrons who did not provide nursing care and were basically housekeepers who oversaw the nurses and maintained order within the hospital. Unlike the nurses, they had to be literate and were usually from a low-middle-class background. The early matrons were ineffective and were not respected by the nurses. This began to change in the midcentury as the doctors called for improved nursing care for their patients. Although nurses did have influence, ultimate control was held by the physician (Helmstadter, 2008).

### Evolution of Nursing Matrons (Helmstadter, 2008)

- Ms. Morterras, matron of the Westminster, 1794–1818: no sense of a nursing system (p. 5)
- Ms. Harris, matron of St. George's Hospital, 1841–1849: a lack of authority and respect (p. 5)
- Ms. Cookesley, matron of the Middlesex, 1835–1849: the need for a supervisor with nursing knowledge (p. 6)
- Ms. Nelson, matron of the London Hospital, 1833–1867: the limitations of a competent old-style matron (p. 7)
- Lady Superintendent Sister Mary Jones, matron of Kings College Hospital, 1856–1868, and Charing Cross Hospital, 1866–1868: religious discipline, respect for the working-class nurses, and centralizing reform (p. 7)
- Florence Nightingale: a failure to gain control of the Nightingale Nursing School (p. 9)
- Flora Masson, matron of the Radcliffe Infirmary, 1891–1897: true nursing spirit and decorum versus increased hospital revenues and dances in the children's ward (p. 10)

## HOSPITALS AND NURSING IN THE 19TH CENTURY

### United States

The Industrial Revolution had a major influence on the nursing profession, with nursing transitioning from unskilled to skilled (Miller, 2006). The Civil War also played a significant role in the continued development of the nursing profession (Miller, 2006). During the first part of the 19th century, many new hospitals were built, and most followed the block design of the Pennsylvania Hospital, Massachusetts

General Hospital, and New York Hospital that were built during the 18th century. In the 1850s, Massachusetts General Hospital took the lead in redesigning hospitals in an effort to lower the incidence of infections and gangrene. Nursing care during this time varied widely, with hospitals run by religious orders providing high-quality care (Rosenberg, 1977).

### *Highlights*

**1813**—Ladies Benevolent Society of Charleston, South Carolina, organized home care for poor Whites and free Blacks

**1817**—The Friends Asylum was established by the Quaker community for the "moral care" of psychiatric patients

**1846**—Anesthesia was used successfully during surgical procedures

**1861**—Dorothea Dix was appointed superintendent of Union Army nurses during the Civil War (Chambers & Subera, 1997)

**Fast Facts in a Nutshell**

In 1839, Joseph Warrington published *The Nurse's Guide*. This guide was developed for nurses who were providing care to mothers and children in the lying-in chamber (now called a maternity ward; Gabrielson, 1976).

### *Civil War*

The American Civil War between the North and South took place between 1861 and 1865 and resulted in significant loss of life both on and off the battlefield (see Exhibit 6.2). Approximately 618,000 troops lost their lives during battle, and for those who survived, many succumbed to their wounds due to a lack of adequately trained physicians and nurses and poor sanitary conditions. Quite notably, Florence Nightingale had a significant positive effect on the health of the British army during the Crimean War and shared her work in her publication, *Notes on Nursing*, which eventually influenced American nurses (Kalisch & Kalisch, 2004).

## London, France, Finland, and Ireland

The hospitals of the early 19th century were vastly different from hospitals at the end of the century. During the latter part of the 19th

Exhibit 6.2

**Civil War Nursing Facts**

- Ten thousand women served (mainly in the North).
- There were 3,214 nurses, appointed by Dorothea Dix, who served as employees of the Union Army (North).
- Nursing care in the Confederate Army (South) was provided mainly by infantrymen, but approximately 1,000 women served as nurses.
- Nursing care was also provided by the Sisters of Charity, Black women employed by General Orders of the War Department, women who performed menial tasks, and volunteers who were not compensated. (Kalisch & Kalisch, 2004; MacLean, 2006; Sheehy, 2007)

century, there was a much greater emphasis on public health and the control of epidemics with the use of isolation and improved sanitary conditions. Quite notably, the shift in hospital construction was greatly influenced by Florence Nightingale and Jacques Tenon, with new hospitals being built across Europe that were considered to have a modern curative design (Allan, 2013).

### *Highlights*

- The London Bible and Domestic Female Mission was founded by Ellen Ranyard in 1857.
- Bible-women nurses provided care to the poor in London.
- The Institute of Nursing Services was created (Denny, 1997).

### *The Crimean War*

The Crimean War took place from 1853 to 1856 with an alliance of Britain, France, Turkey, and Sardinia against Russia for control over the Middle East. In 1854, Sidney Herbert, who was the British secretary of war, sent Florence Nightingale to care for the wounded military in a hospital in Scutari. She brought a contingent of 38 nurses and was horrified at the unsanitary conditions. She believed that the most important issues to address were diet, dirt, and drains, so she focused on cleanliness, ventilation, and good nutrition. She worked tirelessly day and night and was called the "Lady with the Lamp" and "ministering angel" (Cook, 1913, as cited in Fee & Garofalo, 2010, p. 1591).

**Fast Facts in a Nutshell**

During the Crimean War, more soldiers died of typhus, typhoid, cholera, and dysentery than of their wounds from battle (Fee & Garofalo, 2010).

### *Asylum Nursing in London*

The 1845 Lunacy Act in England was something of a turning point in the care of the mentally ill. Prior to this, insane patients were not distinguished from deviant individuals. The Lunacy Act supported the humane treatment of the mentally ill, who were physically and symbolically isolated from other patients and treated by "mad doctors" (Symonds, 1995).

## France

There was a major shift in the provision of health services in Paris from private religious to large public institutions. Physicians provided ward care, studied the pathology of diseases, and were salaried (Allan, 2013).

**Fast Facts in a Nutshell**

Sister Mary Joseph Croake was an Irish Sister of Mercy who served during the Crimean War from 1854 to 1856. She chronicled her patient care experiences during the war and is credited with grounding their nursing according to rights and not privileges. She is credited, along with her fellow nursing Sisters, with setting down the roots of modern nursing and the 19th century's female-led humanitarian movement (Doona, 1995).

## Australia and Queensland

During the 19th century, Australia was a patriarchal country, and nurses were subservient to doctors. Nurses were appointed by doctors, and many were reformed convict women. Australia was unique in that there were many remote areas and a greater population of men (Yuginovich, 2000).

### *Highlights*

Nurses in Australia were:

- Predominately female, and subservient to husbands and doctors
- Practicing in remote areas
- Skilled in home remedies (Yuginovich, 2000)

Key events during this era included the following:

- Royal Brisbane Hospital provided training for country nurses (1826).
- Rules governing nursing were implemented in Queensland (1854).
- An 18-month nurse-training program was provided by Dr. Jackson (1854).
- The first order of Roman Catholic nuns from Dublin arrived in Brisbane (1861).
- Charitable hospitals were developed throughout Queensland (1861).
- Bush nursing originated in Victoria, and nurses provided care to people living in remote areas of Australia and Queensland (Yuginovich, 2000).

## SUMMARY

The nursing profession changed dramatically throughout the 1800s with the advent of formalized nursing schools, more stringent eligibility rules, increases in the number of hospitals, and advances in medicine and science. Many of these changes were influenced by urbanization, industrialization, the Crimean and Civil Wars, and the expanding population.

### Further Reading

Fealy, G., McNamara, M., & Geraghty, R. (2010). The health of hospitals and lessons from history: Public health and sanitary reform in the Dublin hospitals, 1858–1898. *Journal of Clinical Nursing, 19*(23/24), 3468–3476. doi:10.1111/j.1365-2702.2010.03475.x

Helmstadter, C. (1993). Old nurses and new: Nursing in the London teaching hospitals before and after the mid-nineteenth-century reforms. *Nursing History Review, 1*(1), 43–70.

Helmstadter, C. (1994). The first training institution for nurses: St John's House and 19th-century nursing reform: The impact of St John's House on 19th-century nursing reform . . . part 2. *History of Nursing Society Journal, 5*(1), 3–18.

Massie, L. (1995). The role of women in mental health care in 19th-century England. *International History of Nursing Journal, 1*(2), 39–51.

Mortimer, B. (1997). Counting nurses: Nursing in the 19th-century census. *Nurse Researcher, 5*(2), 31–43.

## References

Allan, K. (2013). 19th-century hospitals and the design revolution. *British Journal of Healthcare Management, 19*(5), 214–215.

Chambers, L. E., & Subera, P. (1997). Nursing history as a tool for development of a professional identity within nursing students. *Journal of Nursing Education, 36*(9), 432–433.

Condon, M.A.B. (2001). *The evolution of nursing care of the normal newborn from 1800 to 2000: From a derived standard of care framework.* (Doctoral dissertation). Adelphi University, Garden City, NY. (Pub. No. 3031324).

Denny, E. (1997). The second missing link: Bible nursing in 19th century London. *Journal of Advanced Nursing, 26*(6), 1175–1182. doi:10.1046/j.1365-2648.1997.00430.x

Detar, J. (2009, November). Linda Richards led the way for American nurses. *Investors Business Daily.* Retrieved from Business Source Complete.

Doona, M. (1995). Sister Mary Joseph Croake: Another voice from the Crimean war. *Nursing History Review, 3*(41), 3–41.

Ellis, H. (2009). Mary Seacole: Self-taught nurse and heroine of the Crimean War. *Journal of Perioperative Practice, 19*(9), 304–305.

Fee, E., & Bu, L. (2010). The origins of public health nursing: The Henry Street visiting nurse service. *American Journal of Public Health, 100*(7), 1206–1207.

Fee, E., & Garofalo, M. E. (2010). Florence Nightingale and the Crimean War. *American Journal of Public Health, 100*(9), 1591. doi:10.2105/AJPH.2009.188607

Gabrielson, R. C. (1976). Two centuries of advancement: From untrained servant to skilled practitioner. *Journal of Advanced Nursing, 1*(4), 265–272. doi:10.1111/j.1365-2648.1976.tb00965.x

Hawkins, J., & Watson, J. (2003). Public health nursing pioneer: Jane Elizabeth Hitchcock, 1863–1939. *Public Health Nursing, 20*(3), 167–176.

Helmstadter, C. (2008). Authority and leadership: The evolution of nursing management in 19th-century teaching hospitals. *Journal of Nursing Management, 16*(1), 4–13. doi:10.1111/j.1365-2934.2007.00811.x

Kalisch, P. A., & Kalisch, B. J. (2004). *American nursing: A history* (4th ed.). Philadelphia, PA: Lippincott, Williams & Wilkins.

MacLean, M. (2006). Nursing in the Civil War South: Volunteer Confederate nurses. Retrieved from https://www.civilwarwomenblog.com/nursing-in-the-civil-war-south

Miller, N. (2006). *The American Civil War and other 19th-century influences on the development of nursing* (Doctoral dissertation). Available from ProQuest Dissertations and Theses database. (Publication No. 3243878).

Nightingale, F. (1860). *Notes on nursing: What it is and what it is not.* New York, NY: D. Appleton.

Robinson, J. (2004). *Mary Seacole: The most famous Black woman of the Victorian age.* New York, NY: Carroll & Graf.

Rosenberg, C. E. (1977). And heal the sick: The hospital and the patient in 19th century America. *Journal of Social History, 10*(4), 428–447.

Sheehy, S. (2007). U.S. military nurses in wartime: Reluctant heroes, always there. *Journal of Emergency Nursing, 33*(6), 555–563.

Sitzman, K. (2010). Nursing in the United States during the 1800s. In D. M. Judd, K. Sitzman, & M. Davis (Eds.), *A history of American nursing: Trends and eras* (pp. 38–59). Sudbury, MA: Jones & Bartlett.

Symonds, B. (1995). The origins of insane asylums in England during the 19th century: A brief sociological review. *Journal of Advanced Nursing, 22*(1), 94–100. doi:10.1046/j.1365-2648.1995.22010094.x

Wawersik, J. (1997). History of chloroform anesthesia. *Anaesthesiologie und Reanimation, 22*, 144–152.

Wright, D. (1999). Asylum nursing and institutional service: A case study of the south of England, 1861–1881. *Nursing History Review, 7*, 153–169.

Yuginovich, T. (2000). A potted history of 19th-century remote-area nursing in Australia and, in particular, Queensland. *Australian Journal of Rural Health, 8*(2), 63–67.

# II

# Florence Nightingale and Beyond

# 7

# The Lady With the Lamp: Florence Nightingale and Her Effect on the Nursing Profession in the 19th Century

It is common knowledge that Florence Nightingale had a significant impact on the nursing profession: She is often referred to as the founder of modern-day nursing. Nightingale became a nurse despite the objections of her well-to-do family. She played an influential and pivotal role during the Crimean War, and her focus on cleanliness and the environment is credited with saving the lives of many soldiers. She continued to advocate for health and wellness promotion and a formally trained nurse education program for the rest of her life. Nightingale was also a prolific writer and published more than 200 books on nursing and nursing education (Lim, 2014).

**In this chapter, you will learn:**

- Why the Crimean War was a pivotal point in nursing history
- How Florence Nightingale influenced the course of nursing
- The foundations of nursing theory
- When the first schools of nursing opened
- Nightingale's health and wellness promotion

## FLORENCE NIGHTINGALE (1820–1910)

Florence Nightingale was born on May 12, 1820, while her parents were vacationing in Florence, Italy. Her sister, Parthenope, had been born in Naples, Italy, the year before. The Nightingales were a family of wealth and privilege from England. Florence Nightingale's father was originally named William Shore; however, he changed his last name to Nightingale to honor his relative, Timothy Nightingale, who had left him a fortune earned from mining lead ("Nursing Research Online," 2010).

The Nightingale family lived in Derbyshire and spent summers in a cottage in Lea Hurst. Florence and her sister were tutored by their governesses and schooled in the arts (Ayers, 2014). Their father, who had attended Cambridge University, also played a role in their education and envisioned for both sisters a life of aristocracy. However, Nightingale had a different plan, which may have been influenced by the fact that, as a child, she and her family visited the poor people in town. As a teenager, she continued to visit the poor and often donated money, materials, and food (MacQueen, 2007).

Nightingale was described as serious and frequently took notes on social conditions when she traveled with her family. Unlike her sister, Nightingale knew that social conventions were not for her and at an early age expressed a desire to be a nurse. Indeed, she felt that God was calling her to do this. However, during this era, nursing was not considered a respectable profession. Initially, her parents were against this choice and felt it was beneath her social standing (Ayers, 2014). Eventually, they acquiesced, and in 1851, she attended the Institute of Protestant Deaconesses in Kaiserswerth, Germany, where she spent 3 months receiving her foundational nurse training (Kalisch & Kalisch, 2004; MacQueen, 2007). From this point forward, she devoted her life to nursing and served as a clinician, nursing leader, patient advocate, nursing researcher, community servant, and strong proponent of quality nurse training (Ayers, 2014; see Exhibits 7.1 and 7.2).

Florence Nightingale was somewhat of an enigma, and perhaps because of her aristocratic upbringing, she ventured into unchartered territory and spoke her mind. Her chief concern, according to Benedict (1948/2012), was "'What is best for the patient?' Her whole thought was for the sick, their comfort, their cure" (p. 19). Although she embraced research, she also called upon her own clinical experience and practiced what could be called holistic nursing care, considering the environment, the patient, and the importance of nutrition, care, and comfort (Benedict, 1948/2012).

Exhibit 7.1

## Timeline of Events in Florence Nightingale's Life

**1849**—Spent time with the Sisters of Charity in Alexandria, Egypt
**1851**—At 31 years of age completed 3 months of training at the Institute of Protestant Deaconesses
**1853**—Went to Paris to work with several nursing Sisters in Paris
**1853**—Was appointed superintendent of the Establishment of Gentlewomen During Illness (a charitable hospital for governesses)
**1854**—Was appointed "superintendent of the Female Nursing Establishment of the English General Hospital" ("Florence Nightingale," n.d., slide 2)
**1854**—Led a contingent of 38 self-proclaimed nurses
**1856**—Wrote about nursing during the Crimean War
**1860**—Published her famous *Notes on Nursing: What It Is and What It Is Not* ("Florence Nightingale," n.d.).

Exhibit 7.2

## Florence Nightingale Pledge (1893)

I solemnly pledge myself before God and in the presence of this assembly, to pass my life in purity and to practice my profession faithfully. I will abstain from whatever is deleterious and mischievous, and will not take or knowingly administer any harmful drug. I will do all in my power to maintain and elevate the standard of my profession, and will hold in confidence all personal matters committed to my keeping and all family affairs coming to my knowledge in the practice of my calling. With loyalty will I endeavor to aid the physician in his work, and devote myself to the welfare of those committed to my care.

—Lystra E. Gretter and the Committee for the Farrand Training School for Nurses (as cited in "Florence Nightingale Pledge," 2015)

## Fast Facts in a Nutshell

In her famous book *Notes on Nursing,* which was actually written for "women who were in charge of the health of others," Nightingale advocated for both "sanitary" (ventilation, cleanliness, comfort, nutrition) nursing and "handicraft" nursing (dressings and medicine; Nightingale, 1860, as cited in MacQueen, 2007, p. 31).

Accounts conflict as to whether Florence Nightingale practiced nursing after returning from Crimea. According to MacQueen (2007), Nightingale did indeed continue to practice nursing and provided care to many of the villagers and her family. For example, she nursed her mother during an extended illness and, after her mother's death, cared for her sister, Parthenope. However, it is also true that Nightingale, who fell ill with Crimean fever, had a slow recovery, and was often confined to bed for long periods. She died on August 13, 1910 (Sitzman, 2010).

**Fast Facts in a Nutshell**

"In early life, Florence Nightingale was engaged to her first cousin, John Smithurst of Derbyshire, England. Marriage was forbidden by both families, probably on grounds of consanguinity" (Benedict, 1948/2012, p. 19).

## THE CRIMEAN WAR

The Crimean War between France, the Ottoman Empire, Britain, and the kingdom of Piedmont-Sardinia against Russia began in 1853 and ended in 1856 with the Treaty of Paris. During this time, there was a conflict over the religious rights of Christian minorities in the region of the Crimea. The ensuing war resulted in significant loss of life, with many of the deaths related to disease and deprivation (see Exhibit 7.3; Lambert, 2011; Merridew, 2014; Roberts, 2016).

In 1854, Florence Nightingale took a contingent of 38 nurses to serve in a British military hospital in Scutari, Turkey (Garofalo & Fee, 2010). Conditions were deplorable in the British military hospital, and Florence Nightingale did everything in her power to ensure that the environment was clean, supplies were available, and holistic care was provided. Under her leadership, the hospital transitioned from a dirty, vermin-infested building to a well-run hospital (Whyte, 2010). Because she was often the only nurse on duty during the night, she became known as the "Lady with the Lamp" ("Lady with the Lamp," 2007). Nightingale's role in the Crimean War was a turning point for her, and although she was physically debilitated when she returned to London, she continued to have a major influence on nursing and

Exhibit 7.3

**Crimean War Facts**

- October 1853: The Turks declared war on Russia
- 1853–1856:
  - 21,000 British lives lost
  - 95,000 French lives lost
  - 95,000 Ottoman lives lost
  - 140,000 Russian lives lost
- February 1856: The Treaty of Paris ended the Crimean War (Roberts, 2016)

health care. Her tireless efforts during the Crimean War placed her on the world stage and helped her become a legendary figure even before she returned to London (MacQueen, 2007). With her newfound notoriety, Nightingale was able to transform nursing into an "honorable profession" (Whyte, 2010, p. 19).

## FOUNDATIONS OF NURSING THEORY

Florence Nightingale has been described as a pioneer who laid the foundations of philosophical, scientific, and ethical nursing (Frello & Carraro, 2013). Florence Nightingale was a prolific writer, and her writings have served as a foundation for the nursing profession from Nightingale's era to modern-day nursing. According to Selanders (2010), Nightingale's philosophy and teachings were greatly influenced by her belief in God. Although she had a strong belief in God, she also supported religious freedom and fought against discrimination. She firmly believed that all people, regardless of their religious beliefs, had a right to health care.

Nightingale had very strong beliefs in regard to nursing and health care. For example, she believed that nursing was an art and a science, as well as a true calling. She also wrote extensively about the healing environment and that nursing and medicine were two distinct disciplines. Selanders (2010) posits that although Nightingale did not specifically write the paradigm of nursing, she did address each component: person, environment, nurse, and health. Nightingale's model of nursing is a four-step process that includes observation, identification of needed environment alteration, implementation of the alteration, and identification of the current health state (Selanders, 1998,

p. 259). Nightingale's philosophical beliefs have influenced nursing for well over a century, and nurses continue to use her guiding tenets in their professional practice.

**Fast Facts in a Nutshell**

In the 1870s, Nightingale met Linda Richards, the first professionally trained American nurse, who established nurse-training programs in the United States and Japan (Richards, 1911).

## THE FIRST SCHOOLS OF NURSING

During the 19th century, formalized training programs began to emerge, and many were based on the Nightingale Principles of Nursing Education. Prior to this, physicians taught nurse-training school programs. For example, in 1798, Dr. Valentine Seaman developed a nurse-training program for nurses and midwives at New York Hospital (Kalisch & Kalisch, 2004). Nightingale, who valued education for all women, greatly influenced nursing education with her belief that nurses should be taught theoretical and clinical concepts. She proposed that lectures and books were valuable accessories in a nursing program; however, clinical experience was vital (Selanders, 2010).

When Nightingale returned from the Crimean War in 1856, she was given £50,000 in honor of her work (Whyte, 2010). With this support, she developed a formal nursing school called the Nightingale School of Nursing, which opened at St. Thomas's Hospital in London in 1860 (Kalisch & Kalisch, 2004). In 1861, Nightingale funded an embryonic midwifery training project, hoping to reduce maternal mortality (Whyte, 2010, p. 20). In 1872, the New York Training School was opened. It was the first nurse-training school in America modeled after the Nightingale school. A second school, at the New England Hospital for Women and Children, also opened in 1872 under the leadership of Susan Dimock. Although not considered a Nightingale school, this program was based on the Nightingale guidelines because Dimock had met with Nightingale while in Europe (Kalisch & Kalisch, 2004; see Exhibits 7.4 and 7.5).

Exhibit 7.4

**Timeline of Nurse-Training Programs in Late 19th-Century America**

**1863**—Women's Hospital of Philadelphia nurse-training program was founded (Women's Hospital of Philadelphia, 1964).
**1872**—The New England Hospital for Women and Children training program opened (Massachusetts Board of Registration in Nursing, n.d.).
**1872**—The New York Training School opened at New York Hospital (Kalisch & Kalisch, 2004).
**1873**—The Connecticut Training School opened at New Haven State (Cushing/Whitney Medical Library, 2000).
**1873**—The Boston Training School was founded at Massachusetts General Hospital (Massachusetts Board of Registration in Nursing, n.d.).

Exhibit 7.5

**General Admission Criteria for Nurse-Training Programs**

- Female
- Single or widowed
- 25–35 years of age
- No physical defects
- Two character references (Adapted from Kalisch and Kalisch, 2004)

**Fast Facts in a Nutshell**

Linda Richards was the first graduate of the New England Hospital for Women and Children training program, which was led by Susan Dimock, one of the few female American physicians at the time (Holder, 2004).

The development of these early nurse-training programs had a profound effect on nursing as a profession, and by 1880, 15 schools in the United States had enrolled 322 students, 157 of whom graduated (Kalisch & Kalisch, 2004). During this period, other countries were also developing more formalized nurse-training programs.

## NURSE-TRAINING PROGRAMS AROUND THE WORLD

By the mid to late 1800s, nurse-training programs were being established throughout Europe and elsewhere in the world.

- **Ireland**
  **1870s–1880:** Development of nurse-training programs in Dublin Hospital, supported by the Dublin Hospital Society Fund (Wickham, 2001)
- **England**
  **1852:** Nurse training at Great Ormond Street Hospital, London (Historic Hospital Admission Records Project, 2010)
  **1860:** Nightingale School of Nursing at St. Thomas Hospital, London (British Library Collection Items, n.d.)
- **Canada**
  **1874:** First nurse-training program (hospital-based apprenticeship model) established at the General and Marine Hospital in St. Catherine's, Ontario (Kozier et. al., 2014)
- **Thailand**
  **1896:** The School of Lady Midwifery and Nursing Care in Siriraj Hospital (Thaweeboon, Peachpansri, Pochanapan, Senachack, & Pinyopasakul, 2011)
- **Switzerland**
  **1859–1860:** La Source, the world's first secular autonomous nursing school, founded in Lausanne, Switzerland (eight midwifery students admitted; in 1860, seven additional sick-nursing students admitted to the nursing program; Nadot, 2010)

## HEALTH AND WELLNESS PROMOTION: NIGHTINGALE'S DOCTRINE

Nightingale addressed nursing and health and wellness on multiple levels. She posited that the patient should be put in the best condition for health promotion within the patient's environment. Furthermore, the five essential components of optimal healing included a healing environment that ensured:

- Pure air
- Pure water
- Efficient drainage

- Cleanliness
- Light (Swanson & Wojnar, 2004, p. S43)

According to Lim (2014), Nightingale believed that hospitals should be designed with attention to the environment with a pavilion-style design and space that was sanitary and airy. She was vehemently against smoking, and her health doctrines promoted rest, nutrition, and air quality for all.

## SUMMARY

Florence Nightingale was a visionary, advocate, and influencer. She is still a driving force in modern-day nursing. She promoted her beliefs in an effort to promote health and wellness across the spectrum. This chapter provided only a brief insight into her life and workings. Throughout the years, her life and influential works have been the subject of a multitude of articles and books.

### Further Reading

Canadian Nursing History Collection Online. (2015). A brief history of nursing from the establishment of New France to the present. Retrieved from http://www.historymuseum.ca/cmc/exhibitions/tresors/nursing/nchis01e.shtml

Jolley, J. (2007). Now and then: Always nurses. *Paediatric Nursing, 19*(7), 12.

### References

Ayers, K. (2014). How did Florence Nightingale survive being a trauma coordinator? *Journal of Trauma Nursing, 21*(3), 89–92. doi:10.1097/JTN.0000000000000048

Benedict, E. (1948/2012). The constant flame . . . From the archives, three articles that explore the life and legend of Florence Nightingale. *The Canadian Nurse, 108*(5), 18–20.

British Library Collection Items. (n.d.). The Nightingale Home and Training School for Nurses, St. Thomas's Hospital. Retrieved from https://www.bl.uk/collection-items/the-nightingale-home-and-training-school-for-nurses-st-thomass-hospital#sthash.iKDu0HDY.dpuf

Cushing/Whitney Medical Library. (2000, May). *The Connecticut Training School for Nurses and the dispensary.* Retrieved from http://doc1.med.yale.edu/news/exhibits/hospitals/dispensary.html

*Florence Nightingale* [PowerPoint presentation]. (n.d.). Retrieved from https://www.laguardia.edu/mathportfolio/prabha/Bb/maria-nightinangale.ppt

Florence Nightingale pledge. (2015). *South Carolina Nurse, 22*(2), 4.
Frello, A. T., & Carraro, T. E. (2013). Florence Nightingale's contributions: An integrative review of the literature. *Escola Anna Nery, 17*(3), 573–579. doi:10.1590/S1414-81452013000300024
Garofalo, M. E., & Fee, E. (2010). Florence Nightingale (1820–1910): Feminism and hospital reform. *American Journal of Public Health, 100*(9), 1588. doi:10.2105/AJPH.2009.188722
Historic Hospital Admission Records Project. (2010). The early matrons. Retrieved from http://hharp.org/library/gosh/nurses/early-matrons.html
Holder, V. L. (2004, February). From handmaiden to right hand: The infancy of nursing. *AORN Journal, 79*(2), 374–382, 385–390.
Kalisch, P. A., & Kalisch, B. J. (2004). *American nursing: A history* (4th ed.). Philadelphia, PA: Lippincott, Williams & Wilkins.
Kozier, B. J., Erb, G., Berman, A. J., Snyder, S., Buck, M., Yiu, L, & Leesberg Stamler, L. (2014). *Fundamentals of Canadian nursing: Concepts, process, and practice* (3rd ed.). Toronto, ON, Canada: Pearson
Lady with the lamp. (2007, March). *Current Events, 106*(21), 5.
Lambert, A. (2011). The Crimean War. Retrieved from http://www.bbc.co.uk/history/british/victorians/crimea_01.shtml
Lim, F. (2014). Florence Nightingale: Moments of interface between past and present. *American Nurse Today, 9*(5). Retrieved from https://www.americannursetoday.com/florence-nightingale-moments-of-interface-between-past-and-present
MacQueen, J. S. (2007). Florence Nightingale's nursing practice. *Nursing History Review, 15*, 29–49.
Massachusetts Board of Registration in Nursing. (n.d.). *Historical highlights.* Retrieved from http://www.mass.gov/eohhs/docs/dph/quality/boards/nursing/nursing-historical-timeline.pdf
Merridew, C. G. (2014). I. K. Brunel's Crimean War hospital. *Anaesthesia and Intensive Care, 42*, 13–19. Retrieved from https://search-proquest-com.libproxy.adelphi.edu:2443/docview/1548766919?accountid=8204
Nadot, M. (2010). The world's first secular autonomous nursing school against the power of the churches. *Nursing Inquiry, 17*(2), 118–127. doi:10.1111/j.1440-1800.2010.00489.x
Nursing research online: Florence Nightingale's legacy lives on. (2010). *Lamp, 67*(8), 31.
Richards, L. (1911). *Reminiscences of Linda Richards: America's first trained nurse.* Boston, MA: Whitcomb & Barrows.
Roberts, S. (2016). Crimean chronicle. *Military History, 32*, 32–35.
Selanders, L. C. (1998, June). The power of environmental adaptation: Florence Nightingale's original theory for nursing practice. *Journal of Holistic Nursing, 16*(2), 247–263. doi:10.1177/089801019801600213
Selanders, L. C. (2010, May). The power of environmental adaptation: Florence Nightingale's original theory for nursing practice. *Journal of Holistic Nursing, 28*(1), 81–88. doi:10.1177/0898010109360257

Sitzman, K. (2010). Prelude to modern American nursing. In D. M. Judd, K. Sitzman, & M. Davis (Eds.), *A history of American nursing: Trends and eras* (pp. 22–37). Sudbury, MA: Jones & Bartlett.

Swanson, K. M., & Wojnar, D. M. (2004). Optimal healing environments in nursing. *Journal of Alternative and Complementary Medicine, 10*(Suppl 1), S43–S48.

Thaweeboon, T., Peachpansri, S., Pochanapan, S., Senachack, P., & Pinyopasakul, W. (2011). Development of the School of Nursing, Midwifery, and Public Health at Siriraj, Thailand 1896–1971: A historical study. *Nursing & Health Sciences, 13*(4), 440–446. doi:10.1111/j.1442-2018.2011.00654.x

Whyte, A. (2010, January). Relighting the lamp. *Nursing Standard, 24*(18), 18–20.

Wickham, A. (2001). A better scheme for nursing: The influence of the Dublin Hospital Sunday fund on nursing and nurse training in Ireland in the nineteenth century. *International History of Nursing Journal: IHNJ, 6*(2), 26–34.

Women's Hospital of Philadelphia. (1964). *The Woman's Hospital of Philadelphia records.* Retrieved from http://dla.library.upenn.edu/dla/pacscl/detail.html?id=PACSCL_DUCOM_DUCOMWM002

# 8

# The Nursing Profession in the 20th Century

The 20th century was a time of significant growth, turbulence, and transition. The nursing profession continued to grow with the expansion of more formal nurse-training programs. Public health nursing, although not a new concept, came to the forefront. In the late 1800s and early 1900s, the temperance movement (prohibition of alcohol) gathered momentum in the United States, Britain and its English-speaking colonies and dominions, and most of the Nordic countries (Room, 2004, p. 329). Hall (2010) posits that the national alcohol prohibition in the United States between 1920 and 1933, which was focused on decreasing alcoholism and absenteeism from work, was a failed social experiment that created a large black market and increased organized crime. The Great Depression in the 1930s also led to inadequate services, poor health and nutrition, and an increase in suicides. There were two world wars in the first half of the 20th century, and wars in Korea and Vietnam in the latter half of the century. These conflicts increased the need for medical and nursing care and led more women to enter the workforce, especially during the world wars.

**In this chapter, you will learn:**

- How public health nursing evolved
- The genesis of district nursing

(*continued*)

- The influence of World Wars I and II on the nursing profession
- How training programs in nursing continued to develop

## NURSING AT THE TURN OF THE CENTURY

Nursing at the turn of the century was at a crossroads, with new training programs being developed and the role of the nurse still being established. In many countries it was still considered a domestic role. Furthermore, many families did not wish to see their daughters working outside the home (Kalisch & Kalisch, 2004).

## EARLY 20TH-CENTURY NURSING AND HEALTH

The early 20th century in America has been referred to as the Progressive Era in response to the rapid industrialization and expansion that took place in the late 19th century, when there was economic, social, and political reform (Kalisch & Kalisch, 2004). It was also a time of growth and turbulence for many parts of the world, especially Europe and the United States.

Nursing as a profession was still beset by issues, as many untrained women were still being employed as nurses. For example, in Australia, many untrained nurses worked as private-duty nurses. Although increasing numbers of trained nurses were graduating from training programs, untrained nurses continued to staff hospitals, working under the supervision of trained nurses (Madsen, 2005). During this time, there was also a push to regulate the profession by creating nurse registration to separate trained from untrained nurses (Kalisch & Kalisch, 2004). This trend accelerated at the turn of the century, in geographical locations as diverse as South Africa (1891), Natal (1899), New Zealand (1901), and Great Britain (1902; see Exhibit 8.1). In 1901, the International Council of Nurses held its first meeting in Buffalo, New York. The United States took a bit longer to register nurses because each state had to develop its own legislation (Kalisch & Kalisch, 2004).

## PUBLIC HEALTH NURSING

During the 20th century, the U.S. population increased, and many cities were overcrowded, with unsanitary living conditions and the

Exhibit 8.1

**Timeline of Nursing at the Turn of the Century**

**1880s**—Nurse training was provided in South Africa by English nurses organized into Sisterhoods by churches.
**1891**—The Japanese Red Cross created a 3-year training program.
**1891**—Henrietta Stockton established the first state registration for nurses.
**1901**—Grace Neil of New Zealand, one of the original founders of the International Council of Nurses, helped pass her country's Nurse Registration Act.
**1904**—Grace Neil was instrumental in helping pass her country's Nurse Midwife Act.
**1905**—The first training school in Korea opened in a women's hospital in Seoul
**1913**—Dame Alicia Lloyd Still helped set up the College of Nursing in the United Kingdom.
**1915**—A request made by the Siervas de María religious congregation resulted in the credentialing/professional accreditation of Spanish nurses.
**1919**—The Nurses Registration Act established the General Nursing Council in the United Kingdom.

*Source:* Jones (2012).

spread of infectious diseases. Conditions were worse in the cities, especially in tenements, where there was little or no sanitation available (Garb, 2003). To address this alarming situation, many community organizations hired "trained nurses" to care for the sick in their homes (Buhler-Wilkerson, 1993, p. 1778). Public health nursing became more formalized at the turn of the 20th century. Lillian Wald is credited with founding the famous Henry Street Settlement, a nursing organization that provided first aid stations, maternity health conferences, and social activities, among other services, and with coining the term *public health nurse* (Buhler-Wilkerson, 1993, pp. 1778, 1780). Eventually, public health nursing was practiced across the country, and in addition to caring for the sick and poor, these nurses taught about healthy living and disease prevention. According to a report by Edgecombe (2001), public health nursing has been developing along with the public health movement for at least 100 years.

Tuberculosis was a major public health issue in the early 1900s, especially among the poor, who resided in unhealthy environments with crowded living conditions and poor sanitation (King, 2011). Public health strategies were aimed at the development of open-air schools and summer health camps that were focused on improving the overall health of the patients, who were often malnourished, which made them more susceptible. According to Mary Van Zile, RN, "the field supervisor for the New England Division of the American Red Cross" (Van Zile, 1919, as cited in King, 2011, p. 469), the tuberculosis nurse needed broad training to carry out four responsibilities:

- Provide care to the person with tuberculosis and his or her family;
- Provide sufficient support for the family to maintain a normal standard of living;
- Safeguard the community by teaching the patient, family, and community about prevention;
- Educate the public to support efforts to prevent the spread of this disease. (Van Zile, 1919, p. 781, as cited in King, 2011, p. 469)

Public health nursing in England was known as "district nursing" and was greatly influenced by the teachings of Florence Nightingale. According to Nightingale, the district nurse had to be a nurse from a higher class level and complete another 12 months of training. This training took place at St. Thomas Hospital. The nurse was then required to complete 6 months of district nurse training (Edgecombe, 2001).

Public health nursing in Australia dates back to 1902 in Melbourne and Sydney, when council health workers were assigned by the local government to work with mothers and babies in an effort to reduce infant mortality (Keleher, 2000). The major responsibilities of the public health nurse in Australia included the following:

- Improving quality of life, especially of the poor
- Helping patients become self-sufficient
- Surveillance
- Maternal health education
- Promotion of breastfeeding
- Education about hygiene
- Administering vaccinations and immunizations when they became available (Keleher, 2000)

Public health nursing in Canada dates back to the late 1800s, and in 1910, the Canadian Public Health Association was founded. The terms *visiting nurse* and *district nurse* were often used interchangeably when written about in the various nursing journals, but these nurses were always defined as public health nurses. These early public health nurses were part of an elite group that achieved a higher level of education and provided complex care (McKay, 2009).

## WORLD WAR I

Women have always played an integral part in the care of wounded soldiers, and in the early 1900s, this nursing role was more formalized. Multiple articles and books have been written about the wars, and the following is just a brief overview of the wars and the nurses who cared for the wounded. According to Power (2013), during World War I, 22,000 trained nurses volunteered for the "Army Nurse Corps which was the official arm of the Army Medical Corps" (p. 1323). Notably, these nurses were enrolled in the U.S. Army, but they were considered contract workers, had to commit to working until the end of war, had no rank, and were paid $40 per month for their services if they worked in the States and $50 per month if they worked abroad (Power, 2013).

### *Highlights of World War I Nurses*

- Ten thousand American nurses served abroad, mainly in France.
- British and French doctors taught the nurses new techniques in care for critically wounded soldiers.
- Nurses often slept in tents or in unheated barracks.
- When the fighting intensified in 1918, they worked tirelessly with only 2 hours of sleep per day.
- After the armistice was signed, some nurses stayed until all the American soldiers were well enough to travel back home (Power, 2013).

### Fast Facts in a Nutshell

"The few hundred who remained in the Army Nurse Corps after the end of the Great War pressed for reforms. They asked for equal rank and pay to those in the Corps and were granted this in 1923, making it more agreeable to those who joined during World War Two" (Power, 2013, p. 1323).

## WORLD WAR II

World War II began on September 1, 1939, and ended on September 2, 1945. The Axis Powers included Germany, Italy, and Japan. The Allies included Britain, France, Russia, and the United States. This was one of the costliest and deadliest wars, with an estimated death toll of 60 million (O'Neill, 2006). The death and devastation were widespread as this war was fought in multiple countries. Typhus was particularly widespread during this time, and since there were no antibiotics, nurses focused on hygiene, nutrition, hydration, and the delivery of compassionate and expert care (Brooks, 2014).

### *World War II Notable Mental Health Nurses*

Mental health was a major issue on the battlefield and among the wounded, and nurses had to learn new ways to care for soldiers who were traumatized by what they experienced on the battlefield (Silverstein, 2008). The following were two such nurses:

- Lucille Spooner Votta—stationed in the Philippines
- Hildegard Peplau—stationed at the 312th Station Hospital and School for Military Neuropsychiatry for the European Theatre (Callaway, 2002)

**Fast Facts in a Nutshell**

In 1943, the Cadet Nurse Corps was created to increase the number of nurses, and it provided funding for training in public health and psychiatric nursing care (Willever, 1994).

## MILITARY NURSES DURING THE KOREAN AND VIETNAM WARS

Throughout history, wars have affected the nursing profession. According to Hallquist (2005), World War II set the stage for more nurses to work in various roles in the operating room. During the Korean War (1950–1953), there was a shortage of health care providers, so once again, nurses were needed to fulfill these roles. Army nurses performed many functions in the surgical area: triaging wounds, ordering and administering penicillin, suturing, ligating wounds, and initiating blood transfusions (Hallquist, 2005, p. 646).

At the time of the Vietnam War, there was a nurse shortage on the home front that the war further complicated because the military needed more army nurses to care for the wounded soldiers in Vietnam. There were many efforts aimed at recruitment, including the fact that nurses would have officer titles, but the success was limited, which, according to Vuic (2006), may have been related to the antiwar sentiment and the feminine way in which army nurses were portrayed in recruitment advertisements.

## Fast Facts in a Nutshell

Operation Nightingale (1963) was an intensive recruitment effort during the Vietnam War. The Army Student Nurse Program recruited student nurses, who received monthly wages and educational assistance in exchange for "years of active duty service" (Vuic, 2006, p. 115).

## SUMMARY

The 20th century was a time of great growth and development in the nursing profession. It was also a very turbulent time around the world, with a mix of significant industrialization, population growth, poor living conditions, and two world wars. The wars were the driving force in the recruitment and expansion of the role of military nurses. In the United States, events such as Prohibition, the Great Depression, and the Korean and Vietnam Wars also influenced the nursing profession. In the early 1900s, there was a push to regulate the nursing profession, which led to various countries developing formal registration requirements to separate trained from untrained nurses. This chapter provided a brief overview of some of the influential issues in health care and nursing in the 20th century. The following chapters will provide more in-depth information on the role of nursing, with a chronicle of the past 100 years, with regard to education, research, leaders, theorists, politics, health care, and technology.

### Further Reading

Callaway, B. J. (2002). *Hildegard Peplau: Psychiatric nurse of the century*, New York, NY: Springer Publishing.

Cook, R. (2012). Nursing's finest hour: Part 2. Queen's nurses in the First World War. *British Journal of Community Nursing, 17*(8), 388–389.

Hernández Conesa, J., Cayuela Fuentes, P., Beneit Montesinos, J., & González Jurado, M. (2012). Spanish nurses' credentialing in the 20th century. *International Nursing Review, 59*(2), 175–180. doi:10.1111/j.1466-7657.2011.00966.x

While, A. (2014). World War I remembered with reference to district nurse. *British Journal of Community Nursing, 19*(5), 244–247.

### References

Brooks, J. (2014). Nursing typhus victims in the Second World War, 1942–1944: A discussion paper. *Journal of Advanced Nursing, 70*(7), 1510–1519. doi:10.1111/jan.12314

Buhler-Wilkerson, K. (1993). Bringing care to the people: Lillian Wald's legacy to public health nursing. *American Journal of Public Health, 83*(12), 1778–1786. doi:10.2105/AJPH.83.12.1778

Edgecombe, G. (2001). *Public health nursing: Past and future: A review of the literature.* Copenhagen, Denmark: World Health Organization Regional Office for Europe. Retrieved from http://apps.who.int/iris/bitstream/10665/108460/1/E74237.pdf

Garb, M. (2003). Public health then and now. Health, morality, and housing: The "tenement problem" in Chicago. *American Journal of Public Health, 93*(9), 1420–1430.

Hall, W. (2010). What are the policy lessons of national alcohol prohibition in the United States, 1920–1933? *Addiction (Abingdon, England), 105*(7), 1164–1173. doi:10.1111/j.1360-0443.2010.02926.x

Hallquist, D. (2005). Developments in the RN first assistant role: During the Korean War. *AORN Journal, 82*(4), 644–647. doi:10.1016/S0001-2092(06)60033-1

Jones, M. L. (2012). A brief history of the registration of nurses. *British Journal Of Healthcare Assistants, 6*(1), 41–44.

Kalisch, P. A., & Kalisch, B. J. (2004). *American nursing: A history* (4th ed.). Philadelphia, PA: Lippincott, Williams & Wilkins.

Keleher, H. (2000, December). Repeating history? Public and community health nursing in Australia. *Nursing Inquiry, 7*(4), 258–265.

King, M. G. (2011). Four responsibilities of the tuberculosis nurse, circa 1919. *Public Health Nursing (Boston, Mass.), 28*(5), 469–472. doi:10.1111/j.1525-1446.2011.00975.x

Madsen, W. (2005). Early 20th-century untrained nursing staff in the Rockhampton district: A necessary evil? *Journal of Advanced Nursing, 51*(3), 307–313. doi:10.1111/j.1365-2648.2005.03492.x

McKay, M. (2009). Public health nursing in early 20th-century Canada. *Canadian Journal of Public Health, 100*(4), 249–252.

O'Neill, W. L. (2006). *World War II: A student companion.* Oxford, United Kingdom: Oxford University Press.

Power, J.-A. (2013). Courage and medical innovation: The nurses of World War One. *British Journal of Nursing, 22*(22), 1323.

Room, R. (2004). Alcohol and harm reduction, then and now. *Critical Public Health, 14*(4), 329–344.

Silverstein, C. (2008). From the front lines to the home front: A history of the development of psychiatric nursing in the U.S. during the World War II era. *Issues in Mental Health Nursing, 29*(7), 719–737.

Vuic, K. D. (2006). "Officer. Nurse. Woman." Army Nurse Corps recruitment for the Vietnam War. *Nursing History Review, 14*, 111–159.

Willever, H. (1994, May–June). The Cadet Nurse Corps, 1943-48. *Public Health Reports, 109*(3), 455–457.

# III

# Nursing Profession in the 21st Century

# 9

# Shaping the Modern Nursing Profession: Nursing Theorists and Leaders

The past 100 years have been a time of tremendous change and growth in the nursing profession. As nursing became more advanced and nursing education became more formalized, a cadre of nursing theorists/leaders emerged, shaping the profession and helping develop theoretical bases and philosophical beliefs. Most of their theories address the metaparadigm of nursing, which includes the patient, the nurse, health, and the environment, and many build on previous theoretical work. Notably, nursing theories often have received both positive and negative critiques, and various theories have been embraced by academic and service-related organizations, where they often guide the philosophical beliefs and provide a theoretical framework for care.

**In this chapter, you will learn:**

- Contributions of well-known theorists and how they informed or changed nursing practice
- How various leaders contributed to the advancement of the nursing profession
- Social, political, and health issues that influenced nursing
- Feminism and its influence on the nursing profession

## NURSING THEORY AND THEORISTS

Nursing theorists have played a pivotal role in shaping the nursing profession. Some have expanded on the work of earlier theorists; others have developed new theories and ways of thinking that broadened the perspective of the nursing role. Nursing theories can be grouped into four categories, by level: metatheories, grand theories, middle-range theories, and practice theories. The metaparadigm of person, nurse, health, and environment is the phenomenon of concern to nursing educators, leaders, researchers, and scientists (Hunt, 2013).

> The four levels of theory can be depicted as a triangle with the metatheories on the top. Metatheory is broad and abstract and may include purpose, method, and criteria for testing theories in an attempt to explain the meaning of nursing as a science and a profession. They are the overarching theories that guide our research. (Hunt, 2013, p. 152)

Theories are divided into levels, with the grand theories being broad and abstract. Rogers's (1970) Humanistic Science of Nursing is an example of a grand theory. Middle-range theories are frequently used in nursing research, as they are concrete and easier to measure. Kolcaba's (2001) Comfort Theory is an example of a middle-range theory that has been used in various studies (Hunt, 2013). Another well-known middle-range theory is Transition Theory, which was developed by Afif Meleis (Aligood, 2014). Barbara Carper's (1978) Ways of Knowing are considered an epistemology for nursing rather than a theory (Garrett & Cutting, 2015). Carper (1978) described four patterns of knowing in nursing: empirics, moral/ethical knowledge, personal knowing, and aesthetics. Unknowing and sociopolitical were eventually added.

Many nursing programs, in both academia and service, embrace a particular theory to develop their philosophy of nursing, and academic programs develop their theoretical framework based on the work of one or more nursing theorists. Many nursing theorists have influenced the profession of nursing globally.

**Fast Facts in a Nutshell**

According to Comley (1994), "Many nursing models and theories have been formulated over the last half-century in an effort to guide the practice, education and research of nurses" (p. 755).

## Florence Nightingale (1820–1910): Environment Theory

Florence Nightingale, the founder of modern nursing, is also considered the first nursing theorist. Nightingale's theory included several assumptions regarding nursing: Nursing is an art and science; nursing requires an educational base and is distinct from medicine; and nurses must control or alter the environment (see Chapter 7; Nightingale, 1860; Selanders, 2010).

## Virginia Henderson (1897–1996): Need Theory

Virginia Henderson was an influential nursing theorist and leader who was often referred to as the "first lady of nursing" (Nicely & DeLario, 2011, p. 72). In 1960, she developed the following definition of nursing:

> Nursing is primarily assisting the individual (sick or well) in the performance of those activities contributing to health, or its recovery (or to a peaceful death) that he would perform unaided if he had the necessary strength, will or knowledge. It is likewise the unique contribution of nursing to help the individual to be independent of such assistance as soon as possible. (Henderson, 1960, as cited in Watkins, 1996, p. 205)

She also developed a grand theory known as Need Theory that includes three assumptions: Nurses care for patients until they can care for themselves; nurses are willing to serve; and nurses must be educated in the arts and sciences (Rick, 2013).

## Hildegard Peplau (1909–1999): Interpersonal Theory

Hildegard Peplau developed the Interpersonal Relations Model, based on human relations. It focuses on psychodynamic nursing and understanding one's own behavior to help others identify personal challenges. Peplau served as an Army Corps nurse from 1943 to 1945, which gave her an opportunity to work with American and British physicians who specialized in psychiatric medicine. She later used that experience to create a clinical nurse specialist course at Rutgers University, where she taught from 1954 to 1974. She also is credited with creating one of the first graduate nursing courses offered at Columbia University Teachers College in the 1950s (Callaway, 2002).

**Fast Facts in a Nutshell**

Virginia Henderson's Need Theory includes 14 activities to assist patients in healing. For example, the nurse assists the patient with normal breathing, eating, drinking, and elimination of body wastes (Nicely & DeLario, 2011).

### Faye Glenn Abdellah (1919–): 21 Nursing Problems

Faye Glenn Abdellah was deputy surgeon general from 1981 to 1989. Abdellah had a 40-year career as a commissioned officer in the U.S. Public Health Service (Lessing, 2004). Her theory addressed the physical, social, and emotional problems faced by the patient or family and outlined the role and responsibilities of the nurse (Snowden, Donnell, & Duffy, 2010).

### Dorothy Johnson (1919–1999): Behavioral Systems Model

Dorothy Johnson was more concerned with developing a conceptual model for nursing than a theoretical one. In her model, the emphasis is on the individual (Botha, 1989), who is likened to a system with seven subsystems:

- Social bonds
- Food intake
- Excretion
- Dependency
- Aggression
- Achievement
- Sex (Johnson, 1990)

The individual maintains a steady state by adjusting and adapting (Botha, 1989; Nursing Theories, 2011). Botha notes,

> The person is identified as a behavioural system made up of interrelated sub-systems. The actions or behavioural patterns of the total system are efforts to maintain a behavioural system balance while the environmental forces influence the system. Nursing is concerned with the person as a total entity, which would indicate an involvement with all the sub-systems of the behavioural systems. (Botha, 1989, p. 53)

## Martha Rogers (1914–1994): Unitary Human Beings

Martha Rogers, one of the best-known nursing theorists, is credited with developing the Science of Unitary Beings. At New York University, where she taught, many of the nurses who became experts on her legacy were known as Rogerian scholars. Her theory describes human beings as unified wholes who are continually exchanging energy within the environment, which is described as an open system. Rogers viewed open systems as energy fields that are interactive, open, and infinite. She described how energy fields in a pattern change and become more complex and diverse. She also used the term *pandimensional* to describe an energy field that was nonlinear, without space or time (Fawcett, 2015; Wright, 2007).

## Dorothea Orem (1914–2007): Self-Care Model

Dorothea Orem developed the well-known and frequently cited model of Self-Care, in which she described individual activities that must be done to promote well-being. This model grew out of her 40 years of experience and was based on the concept of self-care deficit. The model has three subsystems: self-care deficit, self-care, and nursing systems (Comley, 1994). When an individual is ill and does not have the ability to engage in self-care activities, the nurse assists the patient by supporting, teaching, or providing care (Smith & Parker, 2015).

## Imogene King (1923–2007): Goal Attainment Theory

Imogene King is credited with developing the Goal Attainment Theory. This theory was derived from the interpersonal system and was actually a synthesis of various ideas and nursing work (Hanucharumkul, 1989). According to King's theory, the individual (who brings unique experiences to the table) interacts with the environment (which is an open system). Three systems interact—personal, interpersonal, and society—and the nurse and patient develop goals together (Hanucharumkul, 1989).

### Betty Neuman (1924–): Health Care Systems Model

Betty Neuman viewed the person as a complete system with interrelated parts. Neuman's approach is holistic; she views nursing as being concerned with providing care for the total person and the nurse–patient relationship as collaborative and encompassing personal and professional beliefs (Ross & Bourbonnais, 1985).

### Rosemarie Parse (1924–): Human Becoming Theory

Rosemarie Parse's Human Becoming Theory focuses on quality of life and includes the totality paradigm, which posits that human beings are a combination of factors—spiritual, biological, psychological, and sociological—and the simultaneity paradigm, which holds that each human is a unitary being in continuous mutual interaction with the environment. In this theory, the patient's own perspective is most important (Edwards, 2000; Smith & Parker, 2015).

### Madeleine Leininger (1925–2012): Culture Care Diversity and Universality

Madeleine Leininger is considered the founder of transcultural nursing and is credited with developing the Culture Care and Universality Theory and the Sunrise Model that corresponds with the theory. According to Leininger (2002), nurses should deliver culturally congruent care that is based on cultural values, beliefs, and practices (Leininger, 2002).

### Ida Jean Orlando (1926–2007): Deliberative Nursing Process

Ida Jean Orlando was an associate professor of nursing and director of nursing for the graduate program in mental health psychiatric nursing at the Yale School of Nursing. The research on mental health that she conducted at Yale eventually led to the development of her theory, the Deliberative Nursing Process (Smith & Parker, 2015; Tyra, 2008). In this theory, Orlando focused more specifically on the patient and the role of the nurse, positing that all patients need to be included in the development of the plan of care (Potter & Tinker, 2000; Schmieding, 1990).

### Sister Calista Roy (1939–): Adaptation Model

Roy's Adaptation Model is based on systems theory. The person being described is viewed as a holistic system, which, when faced with illness, will have either a positive adaptive response or a negative ineffective response (Pinheiro de Medeiros et al., 2015). According to Shultz and Hand (2015), "Two key scientific assumptions are as follows: (1) energy is needed to maintain an organizational state and (2) a dysfunction in one system can affect other systems. The philosophical assumptions are derived from humanism and veritivity" (p. 68). This model has been used in multiple nursing studies.

## Jean Watson (1940–): Philosophy and Science of Caring

Jean Watson is well known around the globe for her Philosophy and Science of Caring. Watson's concepts address the metaparadigm of nursing and are based on caring, which she posits is central to nursing. Ten carative factors are identified, which have been revised repeatedly since they were first proposed in 1979 (Cara, 2003). They are the following (Watson, 1988):

- Forming a humanistic–altruistic value system
- Instilling faith–hope
- Cultivating sensitivity to self and others
- Developing a helping–trust relationship
- Promoting expression of feelings
- Using problem solving during care
- Promoting teaching–learning
- Promoting a supportive, protective, or corrective environment
- Assisting with gratification of human needs
- Allowing for existential–phenomenological forces

## Patricia Benner (1942–): From Novice to Expert

Patricia Benner developed a five-stage model of nursing experience through which nurses advance from novice, to advanced beginner, competent, proficient, and finally expert. Her work is well known and widely embraced by the nursing profession (Altmann, 2007).

### Fast Facts in a Nutshell

Silverstein (2003) suggests that nursing theories will continued to be developed as an integrated system of diverse ways of knowing.

## SOCIAL, POLITICAL, AND HEALTH ISSUES THAT INFLUENCED NURSING

Over the past century, nurses' views of nursing have been influenced by myriad internal and external factors. Some of the growth and development was inspired by the nursing theorists and leaders and some by outside factors, such as immigration; population expansion; advances in science, health care, and technology; regulatory and accrediting agencies; and political factors, especially with regard to health insurance.

**Fast Facts in a Nutshell**

Critical social theory can be used as a tool by nurses to focus on the sociopolitical context of health and health care and to highlight ethical ways to practice nursing (Carnegie & Kiger, 2009).

## FEMINISM AND ITS INFLUENCE ON THE NURSING PROFESSION

In the 1970s, the feminist movement began to make progress in advocating for women to become more autonomous and reject the patriarchal system, which is still prevalent in many countries. Emboldened in part by this movement, more nurses in countries such as the United States and England fought for their rights. Many who obtained advanced degrees and assumed leadership positions have helped lead the profession to new heights (Manajlovich, 2007; Sampselle, 1990).

**Fast Facts in a Nutshell**

Manajlovich (2007) stated, "Although the feminist movement of the 1960s did much to bring women in other professions on an equal footing with men, nursing's low status in the health care hierarchy remains" ("Historical Review," para. 2).

## SUMMARY

The nursing profession has experienced significant growth throughout the past 100 years. Much of this growth can be attributed to the nursing theorists/leaders and advances in education, medicine, health care, and technology. This chapter has highlighted the contributions of several nursing theorists/leaders who had a significant impact on the nursing profession.

### References

Aligood, M. R. (2014). *Nursing theorists and their work* (8th ed.). New York, NY: Mosby.

Altmann, T. (2007). An evaluation of the seminal work of Patricia Benner: Theory or philosophy? *Contemporary Nurse: A Journal for the Australian Nursing Profession, 25*(1–2), 114–123. doi:10.5172/conu.2007.25.1-2.114

Botha, M. E. (1989). Theory development in perspective: The role of conceptual frameworks and models in theory development. *Journal of Advanced Nursing, 14*(1), 49–55. doi:10.1111/j.1365-2648.1989.tb03404.x

Callaway, B. J. (2002). *Hildegard Peplau: Psychiatric nurse of the century.* New York, NY: Springer Publishing.

Cara, C. (2003). A pragmatic view of Jean Watson's caring theory. *International Journal for Human Caring, 7*(3), 51–61.

Carnegie, E., & Kiger, A. (2009). Being and doing politics: An outdated model or 21st-century reality? *Journal of Advanced Nursing, 65*(9), 1976–1984. doi:10.1111/j.1365-2648.2009.05084.x

Carper, B. A. (1978). Fundamental patterns of knowing in nursing. *Advances in Nursing Science, 1*(1), 13–24.

Comley, A. (1994). A comparative analysis of Orem's self-care model and Peplau's interpersonal theory. *Journal of Advanced Nursing, 20*(4), 755–760. doi:10.1046/j.1365-2648.1994.20040755.x

Edwards, S. (2000). Critical review of R. R. Parse's *The human becoming school of thought: A perspective for nurses and other health professionals. Journal of Advanced Nursing, 31*(1), 190–196. doi:10.1046/j.1365-2648.2000.01246.x

Fawcett, J. (2015). Evolution of the Science of Unitary Human Beings: The conceptual system, theory development, and research and practice methodologies. *Visions, 21*(1), *10–16.*

Garrett, B. M., & Cutting, R. L. (2015). Ways of knowing: Realism, non-realism, nominalism and a typology revisited with a counter perspective for nursing science. *Nursing Inquiry, 22*(2), 95–105.

Hanucharumkul, S. (1989). Comparative analysis of Orem's and King's theories. *Journal of Advanced Nursing, 14*(5), 365–372. doi:10.1111/j.1365-2648.1989.tb01542.x

Henderson, V. (1960). *Basic principles of nursing care.* Geneva, Switzerland: International Council of Nurses.

Hunt, D. D. (2013). *The new nurse educator: Mastering academe.* New York, NY: Springer Publishing.

Johnson, D. E. (1990). Behavioral System Model. In M. E. Parker (Ed.), *Nursing theories in practice* (pp. 23–32). New York, NY: National League for Nursing.

Kolcaba, K. (2001). Evolution of the mid range theory of comfort for outcomes research. *Nursing Outlook, 49*(2), 86–92.

Leininger, M. (2002). Culture care theory: A major contribution to advance transcultural nursing and practices. *Journal of Transcultural Nursing, 13*(3), 189–192.

Lessing, M. (2004). Up close and personal: Interview with Rear Admiral Faye Glenn Abdellah. *Military Medicine, 169*(11), iii–xi.

Manajlovich, M. (2007). Power and empowerment in nursing: Looking backward to inform the future. *Online Journal of Issues in Nursing, 12*(1). Retrieved from http://www.nursingworld.org/MainMenuCategories/ANAMarketplace/ANAPeriodicals/OJIN/TableofContents/Volume122007/No1Jan07/LookingBackwardtoInformtheFuture.htmlWhile

Nicely, B., & DeLario, G. T. (2011). Virginia Henderson's principles and practice of nursing applied to organ donation after brain death. *Progress in Transplantation, 21*(1), 72–77.

Nightingale, F. (1860). *Notes on nursing: What it is and what it is not.* New York, NY: D. Appleton.

Nursing Theories. (2011). Nursing theorists. Retrieved from http://currentnursing.com/nursing_theory/nursing_theorists.html

Pinheiro de Medeiros, L., da Costa Souza, M. B., Fernandes de Sena, J., Medeiros Melo, M. D., Soares Costa, J. W., & Fernandes Costa, I. K. (2015, January/February). Roy Adaptation Model: Integrative review of studies conducted in the light of the theory. *Revista da Rede de Enfermagem do Nordeste, 16*(1), 132–140.

Potter, M., & Tinker, S. (2000). Put power in nurses' hands: Orlando's Nursing Theory supports nurses—simply. *Nursing Management, 31*(7), 40–41.

Rick, C. (2013). Joining forces: Taking action to serve America's military families—a White House initiative. In K. A. Goudreau & M. Smolenski (Eds.), *Health policy and advanced practice nursing: Impact and implications* (pp. 121–133). New York, NY: Springer Publishing.

Rogers, M. (1970). *Nursing science: Introduction to the theoretical basis of nursing.* Philadelphia, PA: F. A. Davis.

Ross, M., & Bourbonnais, F. (1985). The Betty Neuman systems model in nursing practice: A case study approach. *Journal of Advanced Nursing, 10*(3), 199–207. doi:10.1111/j.1365-2648.1985.tb00513.x

Sampselle, C. (1990). The influence of feminist philosophy on nursing practice. *Journal of Nursing Scholarship, 22*(4), 243–247.

Schmieding, N. J. (1990). An integrative nursing theoretical framework. *Journal of Advanced Nursing, 15*(4), 463–467. doi:10.1111/j.1365-2648.1990.tb01840.x

Selanders, L. C. (2010, May). The power of environmental adaptation: Florence Nightingale's original theory for nursing practice. *Journal of Holistic Nursing, 28*(1), 81–88. doi:10.1177/0898010109360257

Shultz, S., & Hand, M. W. (2015). Usability: A concept analysis. *Journal of Theory Construction & Testing, 19*(2), 65–70.

Silverstein, C. M. (2003, January). *Looking back to the future in nursing science development from 1952–2002: A historical perspective* (Doctoral dissertation). Retrieved from WorldCat (3091294).

Smith, M. C., & Parker, M. E. (Eds.). (2015). *Nursing theories & nursing practice* (4th ed.). Philadelphia, PA: F. A. Davis.

Snowden, A., Donnell, A., & Duffy, T. (2010). *Pioneering theories in nursing.* Luton, Bedfordshire, United Kingdom: Mark Allen Group.

Tyra, P. A. (2008). In memoriam: Ida Jean Orlando. *Journal of the American Psychiatric Nurses Association, 14*(3), 231–232.

Watkins, M. (1996). Virginia Henderson's contribution to nursing. *Journal of Clinical Nursing, 5*(4), 205.

Watson, J. (1988). *Nursing: Human science and human care: A theory of nursing.* Sudbury, MA: Jones & Bartlett.

Wright, B. (2007). The evolution of Rogers' science of unitary human beings: 21st-century reflections. *Nursing Science Quarterly, 20*(1), 64–67.

# 10

# Pioneers in Nursing Education and Social Activism: Lavinia Lloyd Dock, Isabel Hampton Robb, and Mary Adelaide Nutting

Donna M. Nickitas

From its beginning, nursing was defined as having "charge of the personal health of somebody . . . and what nursing has to do . . . is to put the patient in the best condition for nature to act upon him" (Nightingale, 1860, p. 126). This early definition of nursing was written by Florence Nightingale and represents how strategic she was in her thinking about the importance of the observational skills of the nurse and the impact of the environment on health. Nightingale clearly recognized health promotion and health maintenance as important responsibilities of nursing. As nursing has evolved, it has been strongly influenced by health care policy.

**In this chapter, you will learn:**

- How health policy affects nursing practice
- The roles of nurses in advocacy and social activism

*(continued)*

- The nursing education and social activism of:
  - Lavinia Lloyd Dock
  - Isabel Hampton Robb
  - Mary Adelaide Nutting

## HEALTH POLICY

Health policy affects nurses and patients, whether that policy is created through governmental actions, institutional decision making, or organizational standards. Thus, health policies create a framework that can facilitate or impede the delivery of health care services. The engagement in the process of policy development by nurses is central to creating a health care system that meets the needs of nurses as well as the populations they serve. Several key nurse leaders through nursing history beyond Nightingale have been instrumental in educating and informing nurses about the importance of political activism and a commitment to policy development. One of these key nurse leaders, Lavinia Lloyd Dock, was a nurse, feminist, author, pioneer in nursing education, and social activist. She campaigned for women's suffrage by leading several protests, including picketing at the White House, and was arrested after militant demonstrations in June 1917, August 1917, and August 1918 (American Association for the History of Nursing, 2007). These protest movements for women's rights were instrumental in the 1920 adoption of the 19th Amendment to the U.S. Constitution, granting women the right to vote. Another key policy change that Dock actively influenced was the legislation to allow nurses, rather than physicians, to control their profession.

## PIONEERS IN NURSING EDUCATION

Dock was a contributing editor to the *American Journal of Nursing*, and she authored several books, including (with Mary Adelaide Nutting as coauthor) a four-volume history of nursing and what was for many years a standard nurses' manual of drugs. She received nursing training at the Bellevue Hospital School of Nursing, graduating in 1886 (Ogilvie & Harvey, 2000).

Dock wrote and published (with help from her father and brother) a book on therapeutic medicines in 1890. She campaigned for women's rights for many years (Ogilvie & Harvey, 2000). In 1893, Dock, with the assistance of Isabel Hampton Robb and Nutting, founded the American Society of Superintendents of Training Schools for Nurses of the United States and Canada, which became the National League for Nursing. These nurses advocated for health care policy that addressed issues of social justice and equity in health care, clearly realizing that nurses were potent influencers in policy formation (Ogilvie & Harvey, 2000). Their capacity to analyze the policy process and their ability to engage in politically competent action provided a critical interface between practice, research, and policy (Connolly, 1998).

### Fast Facts in a Nutshell

Dock was an assistant superintendent at Johns Hopkins School of Nursing under Isabel Hampton Robb. With Robb and Mary Adelaide Nutting, she helped found the organization that would become the National League for Nursing (Philips, 1999).

Dock, Robb, and Nutting understood how clinical practice was derived from regulations, laws, and policies, all of which are within the domain of government. They learned about government and regulatory agencies as well as how these bodies influence professional nursing, health care, and public policies (Philips, 1999). With this goal in mind, nurses of today must appreciate this historical effort and work with key policy makers to promote crucial conversations about economic and social policies that can cost-effectively promote the health of communities.

## ADVOCACY AND SOCIAL ACTIVISM

To be successful in leading change in nursing and health care, nurses must know firsthand how to trip the levers for change through advocacy and social activism. As the largest segment of the health care workforce in the United States, nurses are the professionals who spend the most time providing direct care to patients. Armed with the full knowledge and appreciation of the contribution that nurses provide to society overall, nurses play an essential role in advancing the nation's health (Nickitas, 2016). Dock, Robb, and Nutting were nurse leaders who were committed to long-term careers that strengthened nursing education and brought transformational change to nursing and health care (Connolly, 1998). Their legacy has contributed to a strong educational infrastructure that will sustain nursing education for the ages.

### Fast Facts in a Nutshell

The U.S. government spends $2.7 trillion on health care annually (Hartman, Martin, Benson, Catlin, & National Health Expenditure Accounts Team, 2013).

Today, nurse educators are seeking to advance the recommendation in the Institute of Medicine (2010) report, *The Future of Nursing: Leading Change, Advancing Health,* to double the number of U.S. nurses with doctoral degrees by building a well-prepared cadre of researchers, leaders, and practitioners. Currently, fewer than 1% of the nursing workforce has a PhD in nursing or a related field, and a large proportion of nurses are nearing retirement. Nurses with doctorates are needed to educate future generations of nurses. To get the right numbers, there must be competitive salary and benefit packages available so that highly qualified academic and clinical nurse faculty are recruited and retained (Nickitas & Feeg, 2011).

Nickitas and Feeg (2011) write, “Doctorally prepared nurses are well positioned to lead change and advance health care in America. They stand ready to conduct research that becomes the basis for improvements in nursing science and advanced practice” (“Getting It Right,” paras. 1–2). Nursing care is a critical factor in care delivery, and nurses have a pivotal role in meeting evolving health needs of individuals, families, and communities by coordinating that care. The coordination of health care needs and activities is essential to speed recovery, economize on resources, and enhance patient satisfaction. Importantly, nurses have an innate ability to work closely with patients and family caregivers to encourage them and to help patients understand their treatment so that they may actively participate in their own care.

Our nation’s health care system is facing significant challenges. The nurses of tomorrow must be prepared to engage in knowledge and scientific discovery, successfully maneuver in health and public policy, create innovative care delivery models, and be present in the boardrooms in health care, business, and government. The only sure way to increase nursing's influence on health policy and quality improvement is by securing a seat at the table. Nurses can no longer wait to be asked to participate; they must actively recruit and ask others to assist them in gaining access to positions of influence. Nurses are well positioned to drive strategies that affect cost, quality, and safety because they confront these issues every day. They must learn to reach across the aisle to colleagues in all types of public and private organizational and health care settings. It does not matter if your workplace is the bedside or boardroom, classroom or clinic, executive suite or dean's office—each of us is confronted with meeting the daily challenges and priorities of nursing.

## SUMMARY

Throughout history, pioneers have made significant contributions to the profession. Many nurses are familiar with the important work of Florence Nightingale. However, there have been countless others. Lavinia Lloyd Dock, Isabel Hampton Robb, and Mary Adelaide Nutting are three pioneers and social activists who left their mark on our profession.

### References

American Association for the History of Nursing. (2007). *Lavinia Lloyd Dock, 1858–1956*. Retrieved from http://www.aahn.org/gravesites/dock.html

Connolly, C. A. (1998). Hampton, Nutting, and rival gospels at The John Hopkins Hospital and Training School for Nurses, 1889-1906. *Journal of Nursing Scholarship, 30*(1), 23–29.

Hartman, M., Martin, A. B., Benson, J., Catlin, A., & National Health Expenditure Accounts Team. (2013). National health spending in 2011: Overall growth remains low, but some payers and services show signs of acceleration. *Health Affairs, 32*(1), 87–99. doi:10.1377/hlthaff.2012.1206

Institute of Medicine. (2010). *The future of nursing: Leading change, advancing health*. Washington, DC: National Academies Press.

Nickitas, D. M. (2016). Economics and populations primary care. In S. B. Lewenson & M. Truglio-Londrigan (Eds.), *Practicing primary health care in nursing: Caring for populations* (pp. 75–88). Burlington, MA: Jones & Bartlett.

Nickitas, D. M., & Feeg, V. (2011). Doubling the number of nurses with a doctorate by 2020: Predicting the right number or getting it right? *Nursing Economics, 29*(3), 109–125.

Nightingale, F. (1860). *Notes on nursing: What it is, and what it is not*. New York, NY: D. Appleton.

Ogilvie, M., & Harvey, J. (Eds.). (2000). *The biographical dictionary of women in science: Pioneering lives from ancient times to the mid-twentieth century.* New York, NY: Routledge.

Philips, D. (1999). Healthy heroines: Sue Barton, Lillian Wald, Lavinia Lloyd Dock and the Henry Street Settlement. *Journal of American Studies, 33*(1), 65–82. doi:10.1017/S0021875898006070

# 11

# The Growth of Nursing Education and Expansion of Degree Programs

*I may be compelled to face danger, but never fear it, and while our soldiers can stand and fight, I can stand and feed and nurse them.*
—Clara Barton

The training and education of nurses around the world changed radically after Florence Nightingale opened the first school of nursing. Although there were training programs prior to this time, training was often provided informally on an individual mentoring basis or by physicians (Kalisch & Kalisch, 2004). Although there was overlap in the development of the various programs, the basic progression of formalized nurse generalist education is (a) formal training programs, (b) registered nurse diploma programs, (c) associate degree programs, and (d) baccalaureate degree programs. "Nursing is one of a few professions that have multiple educational paths for entry into practice" (Spetz & Bates, 2013, p. 1859). Today, nurses can select the diploma, associate degree, or baccalaureate pathway. Currently, there is a push to increase the number of baccalaureate-prepared nurses.

**In this chapter, you will learn:**

- Landmark reports that influenced nursing and the evolution of training schools

*(continued)*

- How the development of diploma programs, associate degree programs, and baccalaureate degree programs evolved
- Why nurses supported advanced degrees in master's and doctoral programs
- Current trends resulting in the expansion of nurse practitioner programs
- The requirements of licensure
- How nurse education in the United States compares with that in other countries

## LANDMARK REPORTS

Nursing education programs have been influenced by many factors, and several reports have been most influential in advancing the profession (see Exhibit 11.1). In the early 1900s, the Rockefeller Foundation sponsored a meeting to discuss the education of public health nurses.

Exhibit 11.1

### Timeline of Important Events in Nursing Education

**1910**—Teachers College, Columbia University, offered the first university postgraduate training program for nurses in nursing education ("What Women Are Doing," as cited in Steedman, 2011).

**1912**—The National Organization for Public Health Nursing was founded to establish services for the new role of the public health nurse (University of Pennsylvania School of Nursing, n.d.).

**1919**—Josephine Goldmark was appointed secretary of the Committee on Public Health Education (Goldmark, 1923).

**1922**—The national nursing honor society, Sigma Theta Tau, was founded at Indiana University (Barron McBride, 2016).

**1923**—The Goldmark report, *Nursing and Nursing Education in the United States,* resulted from a meeting sponsored by the Rockefeller Foundation that focused on the state of public health nursing and required education (Goldmark, 1923).

**1928**—The Burgess report, *Nurses, Patients, and Pocketbooks,* was published.

**1948**—The Brown report, *Nursing for the Future,* was published; its genesis—resulting from a serious nursing shortage after World War II—also prompted the Carnegie Foundation to commission Dr. Esther Lucille Brown to investigate the education of nurses (American Association of Colleges of Nursing, n.d.).

**1948**—The Committee on the Function of Nursing recommended that licensed practical nurses be trained at the associate level and registered nurses be trained at the bachelor's level (Barron McBride, 2016).

**1952**—Fairleigh Dickinson University opened the first associate degree program for nurses (Barron McBride, 2016).

However, the committee soon realized that it also needed to study general nurse education. The Goldmark report (Goldmark, 1923) recommended that all well-rounded nurses have experience in public health nursing. It also called for the strengthening of university programs with an emphasis on nursing leadership and the need for an endowment for nursing education. Following this report, May Ares Burgess was commissioned to study the state of nursing, nursing education, and economics. In her published report, Burgess (1928) posited that nurses should assist the patient toward health and that there was a great need for improvements in education (as cited in Rutherford, 2012). The Brown report (Brown, 1948) recommended that nurses be educated in colleges and universities and that practical nurses receive vocational training. Certainly there have been other reports; however, these were some of the most influential ones.

### Fast Facts in a Nutshell

The Nurse Training Act (Bolton Act), passed in 1948, established the Cadet Nurse Corps, a government program to expand enrollment and shorten the training period to increase the number of nurses working in the armed forces, government and civilian hospitals, health agencies, and war-related industries (U.S. Cadet Nurse Corps, 2010, as cited in Appalachian State University, n.d.).

## Early Nurse Leaders Who Influenced Nursing Education

During this period, a number of nurse leaders were instrumental in helping standardize and improve the educational requirements for nurses enrolled in training schools.

- Isabel Hampton Robb (1893) proposed a 3-year program in which students would receive a "truly liberal education in exchange for three years of service" (Dolan, 1973, p. 276).

- Mary Agnes Snively (1895) published a paper on uniformity in nursing (Ward, 2010).
- Sophia Palmer (1896) spoke against using student nurses as a means of revenue for hospitals (Ward, 2010).
- "Ethel Gordon Fenwick founded the British Nurses' Association and the *British Journal of Nursing*, serving as its editor for many years. She also founded the International Council of Nursing in 1899" (Dorsey & Schowalter, 2008, p. 13).
- Adeline Nutting supported elevating the standards for admission and education. She also became the first known nurse to chair a university department at Teachers College, Columbia University, in 1907 (Steedman, 2011).
- Martha Jenks Chase (1911) designed the first training mannequin at the request of A. Lauder Sutherland, who was in charge of the Hartford Hospital Training School and felt that student nurses needed laboratory experience to increase their technical skills (Grypma, 2012).
- Dr. Richard O. Beard (1920s) and Robb developed the curriculum for a school of nursing in Illinois (Brozenac, 1991, as cited in Ruby, 1999).
- Isabel Stewart succeeded Nutting as chair of the Department of Nursing Education at Teachers College in 1925. Her publications on nursing influenced nursing for many years (Goostray, 1954).
- Katharine Densford Dreves served as president of the American Nurses Association (1944–1948), second vice president of the International Council of Nurses, and dean of the University of Minnesota School of Nursing (American Nurses Association, n.d.).

## Training Programs

Nurse training prior to the 19th century was often done in an informal manner with on-the-job training and experienced nurses mentoring new nurses. At the turn of the 18th century, in 1798, one notable program was organized by a physician named Valentine Seaman, and a separate program run by the Nurse Society of Philadelphia trained nurses to care for mothers during childbirth and the postpartum period in the early 1800s (Kalisch & Kalisch, 2004). "The period of 1893–1913 was a time of major growth and change. There was a rapid expansion in nursing schools. Accordingly, the number of schools increased from sixty-four to one thousand seven hundred and seventy-six" (Faison, 2012, p. 2). In 1983, the American Society of Superintendents of Training Schools for Nurses, a forerunner of the National

League for Nursing (NLN), was founded; this organization pushed for the establishment of educational standards in nursing training programs (American Commission for Education in Nursing, 2016). The growth of these programs was directly related to the population growth in addition to public health issues, the poor economy, and the world wars.

## Fast Facts in a Nutshell

Howard University, Teachers College, the University of Texas at Galveston, and Rush Medical College were considered the earliest university-level nursing programs, and in 1909 the University of Minnesota "became the first university to have an official school of nursing" (Barron McBride, 2016, "A Brief History," para. 2).

### *Diploma Programs*

Three-year diploma programs served as the mainstay of nursing education in the 20th century. These programs were most often hospital based, and teaching was initially done by physicians and eventually experienced nurses. These programs were offered for 3 years and with a strong concentration of nursing courses. At the inception of the diploma programs, much of the clinical training was based in the hospital where the program was offered, and student nurses worked long shifts as part of their training. However, in accordance with accreditation standards and current guidelines, diploma programs put an end to that practice, although students did receive more clinical training compared to the other programs. According to the survey released by the NLN (2015), there were 67 diploma school programs in the United States in 2014 compared with more than 200 diploma programs in 1986.

### *Associate Degree Programs*

The associate degree programs were introduced in the 1950s in an effort to educate a cadre of nurses to meet the demand for more nurses after World War II. According to Mahaffey (2002), the 2-year associate degree program was introduced in 1952 as a project at Teachers College, Columbia University. Dr. Montag developed the 2-year program, which offered a patient-centered education in community and junior colleges. The project was supported by a grant from the Kellogg

Foundation, and in 1958, these new programs were piloted in seven states. The pilot was a huge success, and these programs were widely embraced and continue to serve as an entry into practice for approximately half of the current nursing workforce. The curriculum was in line with associate degree–level programs, and students had to complete college-level coursework. According to the NLN (2015), in 2014 there were 1,092 associate degree programs in the United States. Although there is currently a greater push for baccalaureate-prepared nurses, at least in some parts of the United States (see Chapter 14), associate degree programs are still very popular, with approximately 60% of the U.S. workforce being prepared at the associate degree level (Spetz & Bates, 2013).

### *Baccalaureate Degree Programs*

Baccalaureate education for nurses has been supported by several nursing leaders since the early 20th century. For example, Fenwick (1901), the founder of the International Council of Nurses, discussed and supported education for nurses at the university level. The Brown report (Brown, 1948) called for nurse training to be at the university level, and the American Nurses Association published a position paper in support of baccalaureate preparation for nurses in 1964. According to the NLN (2015), there were 710 Bachelor of Science in Nursing (BSN) programs in the United States in 2014 in comparison with approximately 420 programs in 1986.

### *Master's Degree Programs*

Prior to the 1950s, nurses who wanted to earn a master's degree had to attend a non-nursing program. However, that changed, and currently there are more than 330 master's degree programs accredited by the Commission on Collegiate Nursing. "A nurse prepared at the master's level also is clearly able to serve important functions as an expert clinician as a faculty member in a nursing education program. *However, the primary focus of the master's education program should be the clinical role*" (American Association of Colleges of Nursing, 1996, p. 3, emphasis in original).

### *Nurse Practitioner Programs*

Nurse practitioner (NP) programs date back to 1965, when Dr. Loretta Ford and Dr. Henry Silver at the University of Colorado developed the first program. In 1967, Boston College initiated one of the first master's-level NP programs. Since that time, the role, education, and scope of practice for NPs have evolved. In 2013, the Academy of Nurse Practitioners and the American College of Nurse Practitioners joined forces to become the American Association of Nurse Practitioners, and in 2014, there were 192,000 NPs in the United States (American Association of Nurse Practitioners, n.d.), with specialties including family nurse practitioner, acute care nurse practitioner, geriatric nurse practitioner, advanced practice nurse, nurse-midwife, and nurse-anethetist. NP roles and scope of practice continue to be defined, and the Institute of Medicine's (2010) *Future of Nursing Report* has certainly influenced the role of the NP (see Chapter 10).

### *Licensure*

All nurses must pass a licensure exam after they complete their basic nursing program and renew their licenses in accordance with their state or country's education/licensing board. "The year 1903 marked the passage of the first four laws to regulate the practice of nursing in the United States. The first of these to be enacted was signed into law on March 3 by the governor of North Carolina" (Dorsey & Schowalter, 2008, p. 19). Since this time, there have been many changes and advances in the requirements for licensure and practitioner and school certification. A more detailed description can be found in the publication of the National Council of State Boards of Nursing, titled *The First 25 Years: 1978–2003* (Dorsey & Schowalter, 2008).

## DOCTORAL DEGREE PROGRAMS

Doctoral degree programs have been in existence since the Middle Ages, but they became popular in nursing in the 20th century. Initially, nurses had to earn their doctoral degrees in a discipline outside of nursing. Today, multiple options for nurses have led to some confusion, for example, the Doctor of Philosophy (PhD), Doctor of Nursing Science (DNS), and Doctor of Nursing Practice (DNP) degrees. The PhD and DNS degrees are very similar, and some universities have actually changed their DNS degrees to PhD degrees (Reid Ponte & Nicholas, 2015). According to Reid Ponte and Nicholas (2015), "[i]n the past decade, the profession appears to have reached an informal consensus that the PhD is the preferred research-intensive doctoral degree in nursing, and the DNP is the preferred terminal practice degree" (p. 352). Clearly, these programs will continue to be updated to meet the current and future needs of our profession.

The DNP has been in existence since 1979, when it was first offered by Case Western University. However, it was not until around 2004 that it gained popularity and was considered a viable alternative to the research-focused degrees of doctor of philosophy and doctor of nursing science. There has been great controversy and some ambiguity related to this degree, which is considered a practice degree; at one point, the American Association of Colleges of Nursing (n.d.) demanded that all advanced practice nurses earn a DNP by 2015. Due to conflicting views and a lack of consensus, this did not come to pass. According to Terhaar, Taylor, and Sylvia (2016), the demand for DNP-prepared nurses is high, but many programs lack rigor.

**Fast Facts in a Nutshell**

"The National League for Nursing Education, American Association of Collegiate Schools of Nursing, and the American Nurses Association have contributed to the debate to define nursing educational preparation and practice. In the mid-20th century there were two levels of nursing preparation—the professional and technical nurse" (American Association of Colleges of Nursing, n.d., p. 4).

### Nurse Education in China

Nursing in China in the early 1900s was considered a vocational profession. Training was mainly hospital based, and most of the textbooks were in English. In 1951, all nursing programs were standardized to 2 years in length. However, in 1954, they were increased to 3 years, and all curricula included teachings on traditional Chinese medicine and were highly regulated. There have been many positive changes in nursing education, and in 2008, a new Nurse Practice Act placed a greater emphasis on nursing education. Most of the programs today are diploma and baccalaureate, and recently the role of advanced practice nurses has been embraced (Wong & Zhao, 2012).

## SUMMARY

Nursing education has become more standardized and thorough with the creation of multiple levels ranging from diploma to doctoral. Many of these changes came about in response to reports published in the first half of the 20th century. Nursing education will continue to evolve, as the recent increase in NPs and nurses with PhDs shows, and the United States is not the only country experiencing this evolution.

## Further Reading

Zahran, Z. (2012). Nurse education in Jordan: History and development. *International Nursing Review, 59*(3), 380–386. doi:10.1111/j.1466-7657.2011.00947.x

## References

American Association of Colleges of Nursing. (n.d.). Lessons learned from an historical sample of nursing education–practice partnerships compiled by Dr. Martha Mathews Libster. Retrieved from http://www.aacn.nche.edu/downloads/academic-practice-partnerships-task-force/NursingHeritageTable.pdf

American Association of Colleges of Nursing. (1996, March). *The essentials of master's education for advanced practice nursing.* Washington, DC: Author.

American Association of Nurse Practitioners. (n.d.). Historical timeline. Retrieved from https://www.aanp.org/all-about-nps/historical-timeline

American Commission for Education in Nursing. (2016). ACEN and the history of nursing accreditation. Retrieved from http://www.acenursing.org/acen-history-of-accreditation

American Nurses Association. (n.d.). Katharine Densford Dreves (1890-1978) 1984 inductee. Retrieved from http://www.nursingworld.org/KatharineDensfordDreves

Appalachian State University. (n.d.). The beginning of associate degree nursing education in North Carolina. Retrieved from http://www.nursinghistory.appstate.edu/beginnings-associate-degree-nursing-education-nc

Barron McBride, A. (2016). *Professional nursing education—Today and tomorrow.* Washington, DC: National Academic Press. Retrieved from https://www.ncbi.nlm.nih.gov/books/NBK232658

Brown, E. L. (1948). *Nursing for the future: A report prepared for the National Nursing Council.* New York, NY: Russell Sage Foundation.

Burgess, M. A. (Ed.). (1928). *Nurses, patients, and pocketbooks: Report of study of the economics of nursing conducted by the Committee on the Grading of Nursing Schools.* New York, NY: Garland.

Dolan, J. (1973). *Nursing in society: A historical perspective* (13th ed.). Philadelphia, PA: W. B. Saunders.

Dorsey, C. F., & Schowalter, J. M. (2008). *The first 25 years: 1978–2003.* Chicago, IL: National Council of State Boards of Nursing.

Faison, K. (2012). Nursing education: A historical overview. *JOCEPS: The Journal of Chi Eta Phi Sorority, 56*(1), 2–4.

Fenwick, E. J. (1901). *The organization and registration of nurses.* Proceedings of the Third International Congress of Nurses, Buffalo, NY.

Goldmark, J. (1923). *Nursing and nursing education in the United States: Report of the Committee for the Study of Nursing Education.* New York, NY: Macmillan.

Goostray, S. (1954). Isabel Maitland Stewart. *American Journal of Nursing, 54*(3), 306–307.

Grypma, S. (2012). Regarding Mrs. Chase. *Journal of Christian Nursing, 29*(3), 181.

Institute of Medicine. (2010). *The future of nursing: Leading change, advancing health.* Washington, DC: National Academies Press.

Kalisch, P. A., & Kalisch, B. J. (2004). *American nursing: A history* (4th ed.). Philadelphia, PA: Lippincott, Williams & Wilkins.

Mahaffey, E. H. (2002). The relevance of associate degree nursing education: Past, present, future. *Online Journal of Issues in Nursing, 7*(2). Retrieved from http://www.nursingworld.org/mainmenucategories/anamarketplace/anaperiodicals/ojin/tableofcontents/volume72002/no2may2002/relevanceofassociatedegree.Aspx

National League for Nursing. (2015). Nursing programs 2013–2014. Retrieved from http://www.nln.org/newsroom/nursing-education-statistics/nursing-programs

Reid Ponte, P., & Nicholas, P. K. (2015). Addressing the confusion related to DNS, DNSc, and DSN degrees, with lessons for the nursing profession. *Journal of Nursing Scholarship, 47*(4), 347–353. doi:10.1111/jnu.12148

Ruby, J. (1999). History of higher education: Educational reform and the emergence of the nursing professorate. *Journal of Nursing Education, 38*(1), 23–27.

Rutherford, M. M. (2012). Nursing is the room rate. *Nursing Economics, 30*(4), 193–200, 206.

Spetz, J., & Bates, T. (2013). Is a baccalaureate in nursing worth it? The return to education, 2000–2008. *Health Services Research, 48*(6, Pt. 1), 1859–1878. doi:10.1111/1475-6773.12104

Steedman, E. J. (2011, August). Mary Adelaide Nutting (1858–1948). Retrieved from http://msa.maryland.gov/megafile/msa/speccol/sc3500/sc3520/013500/013593/html/13593bio.html#35

Terhaar, M. F., Taylor, L. A., & Sylvia, M. L. (2016). The doctor of nursing practice: From start-up to impact. *Nursing Education Perspectives, 37*(1), 3–9. doi:10.5480/14-1519

University of Pennsylvania School of Nursing. (n.d.). Nursing through time: 1900–1929. Retrieved from http://www.nursing.upenn.edu/nhhc/nursing-through-time/1900-1929

Ward, F. (2010). A road not taken: The proposal for a Harvard School of Nursing. *Nursing Inquiry, 17*(2), 128–141.

Wong, F. Y., & Zhao, Y. (2012). Nursing education in China: Past, present and future. *Journal of Nursing Management, 20*(1), 38–44. doi:10.1111/j.1365-2834.2011.01335.x

# 12

# Nursing Research: Quantitative and Qualitative Research and Using the Evidence in Practice

*As knowledge increases, wonder deepens.*

—Charles Morgan

All disciplines require a body of scientific knowledge that is based on research and evidence. Although nurses have been caring for patients for thousands of years, the turning point of professional nursing is often attributed to Florence Nightingale. During the Crimean War, Nightingale collected and analyzed data on the war and recommended that nurses undertake systematic inquiry (University of Maryland School of Nursing, n.d.-b); however, it took about 50 years for nurses to begin formal research (University of Maryland School of Nursing, n.d.-a). Today, there is a great emphasis on scientific inquiry, research, and evidence-based practice and the continued development of nursing's body of scientific knowledge.

**In this chapter, you will learn:**

- How research from other disciplines influences nursing
- The scope of nursing research
- What is meant by quantitative inquiry

(*continued*)

- What is meant by qualitative inquiry
- How evidence-based practice derives from research
- The role of professional journals in advancing nursing
- How the National Institute of Nursing Research supports nursing practice

## RESEARCH FROM OTHER DISCIPLINES

As nursing has evolved over the past 100 years, particularly since the 1950s, the profession has sought to systematically develop its own body of knowledge. Initially, nurse researchers used theories from other disciplines. Kukkala and Munnukka (1994) note that many of these theories were adapted and molded to better suit nursing's phenomena of concern. For example, several early researchers developed nursing theories based on the Need Theory, which originated in psychology. Among them were Abdellah, Henderson, Orem, and Roper (in Europe). (For a comprehensive discussion of nursing theorists, see Chapter 9.) Later, nursing researchers used knowledge that was "sought from existentialism, phenomenology, psychology, sociology and education" (Kukkala & Munnukka, 1994, p. 322).

Since the 1950s, there has been continued development of nursing research, with nurses initially following a positivist model of quantitative research, then moving on to qualitative research, until today's focus on evidence-based practice.

**Fast Facts in a Nutshell**

The essence of a discipline is its body of scientific knowledge, its system of values and ethics, and its societal worth. In a practice discipline such as nursing there is the added dimension of thoughtful and discriminating application of knowledge from other disciplines and perspectives (Carper, 1978). It is this complex relationship between the building of a body of science, the utilization of knowledge from multiple disciplines, and the application to practice and health policy that presents opportunities and challenges for the academic nursing community.
(American Association of Colleges of Nursing, 2006, p. 12)

## NURSING RESEARCH

We live in a complex, ever-changing society that requires multiple perspectives, and interdisciplinary collaboration is an essential characteristic of nursing research that is required for the complex study of health and illness experiences of society (American Association of Colleges of Nursing, 2016). "A discipline attains its social legitimacy, in part, through its ability to demonstrate its contribution to society, not in the here-and-now, but over time" (Fealy, Kelly, & Watson, 2013, p. 1882).

The scientific body of nursing knowledge has continued to grow at a steady pace since the 1950s, as nursing theorists and leaders realized the importance of developing their own body of knowledge. Although nursing knowledge overlaps with that of other disciplines, it is also vastly different, as its focus is holistic and based on health and wellness promotion, as well as caring. In the 1950s, nurse researchers began to study nursing education, their own attitudes and relationships with other health professionals, and patient care. Many of these studies were grounded in sociology, anthropology, and psychology and avoided the medical model to establish nursing as a distinct discipline (Sarkas & Connors, 1986). Education also played a reciprocal role in nursing research; as more nurses earned their graduate degrees, there were more nurse researchers, which increased the number of studies. National nursing organizations also contributed to the body of research. In the 1950s, the American Nurses Association conducted a 5-year study on nursing and later used the findings to guide the development of qualifications and standards for nurses and the profession (Grove, Gray, & Burns, 2014). Since the 1970s, there has been a dramatic increase in the number of nursing studies, with many of them addressing various clinical issues (see Exhibit 12.1).

Exhibit 12.1

### Timeline of Significant Events in Nursing Research

**1952**—*Nursing Research* was the first journal to publish nursing research (*Nursing Research* staff, 1952).

**1979**—The *Western Journal of Nursing Research* was published (Brink, 1979).

**1986**—The National Center for Nursing Research was established to support and fund nursing research (National Institute of Nursing Research [NINR], n.d.).

**1991**—*Qualitative Health Research* premiered (Morse, 1991).

(*continued*)

Exhibit 12.1

**Timeline of Significant Events in Nursing Research (*continued*)**

**1993**—The National Center for Nursing Research was renamed the National Institute of Nursing Research to expand funding for nursing research (NINR, n.d.).
**2007**—Quality and Safety Education for Nurses competencies were published (Cronenwett et al., 2007).
**2010**—The Institute of Medicine released its report, *The Future of Nursing* (Institute of Medicine, 2010).

Myriad factors have influenced nursing research in the past 100 years, and research has made it possible to place a greater emphasis on evidence-based practice.

**Fast Facts in a Nutshell**

The Agency for Healthcare Research and Quality encouraged evidence-based practice in 1997 by creating 12 centers in the United States and Canada dedicated to producing evidence-based reports (Grove et al., 2014).

## QUANTITATIVE RESEARCH

Beginning with the work of Nightingale, early nursing researchers frequently conducted quantitative research, which is grounded in positivism and based on the scientific method. Quantitative research may be used to test the effectiveness of an intervention, test a theory, or test whether a cause-and-effect relationship exists. Quantitative research is further broken down into experimental, quasi-experimental, and nonexperimental (Hunt, 2015). Although many nurse researchers continue to conduct quantitative research, in the 1980s there was a shift to conducting more qualitative research (Grove, Gray, & Burns, 2014).

## QUALITATIVE RESEARCH

Since the 1990s, qualitative research has been widely embraced by nursing researchers (Grove et al., 2014). There are five types of qualitative research: grounded theory, phenomenology, ethnography, historical method, and case study design. Qualitative research often has been viewed with skepticism, with researchers having to justify their approach and findings. However, qualitative research provides rich data, providing nurses a greater understanding of a particular phenomenon in relation to the human experience (Hunt, 2015).

## EVIDENCE-BASED PRACTICE

Recently, evidence-based practice has been widely embraced by the nursing profession along with the rest of the interprofessional team, especially in light of its positive outcomes. According to Eastbrooks (2004), the evidence-based practice movement can be traced back to the United Kingdom–based Royal College of Nursing in the 1960s, when researchers studied the clinical effectiveness of nursing care. However, recently evidence-based practice has become the gold standard in patient care research (Grove et al., 2014). Evidence-based practice has three main tenets: a systematic review of available studies, clinical expert opinion, and inclusion of patient values (Hunt, 2015). Once a review of the available research literature is conducted, the expert team of interprofessional researchers reaches a conclusion as to whether there is enough evidence to develop a protocol or guideline; if not, a recommendation for further research is made.

## HIGHLIGHTS OF PROFESSIONAL JOURNALS: INITIAL PUBLICATIONS

Today, there are a plethora of professional nursing journals, but in the early 1900s, there were only a few. Most professional organizations also publish monthly or bimonthly journals. The following is a select list of some influential journals that were initially published in the 1900s:

**1900**—*American Journal of Nursing*
**1952**—*Journal of Nursing Research*
**1962**—*Journal of Nursing Education*
**1967**—*Journal of Nursing Scholarship* (original title: *Sigma Theta Tau Journal*)
**1976**—*Journal of Advanced Nursing*

**1979**—*Western Journal of Nursing Research*
**1985**—*Journal of Professional Nursing*
**1998**—*Evidence-Based Nursing*

## NATIONAL INSTITUTE OF NURSING RESEARCH

The NINR (established in 1993) has played an influential role in the ongoing development and support of nursing research through its leadership and various grants available to nursing researchers (NINR, 2014). Its website provides brochures and training videos, among other resources.

### Fast Facts in a Nutshell

**NINR Mission Statement:** The mission of the NINR is to promote and improve the health of individuals, families, and communities. The institute supports and conducts clinical and basic research and research training on health and illness across the life span to build the scientific foundation for clinical practice, prevent disease and disability, manage and eliminate symptoms caused by illness, and improve palliative and end-of-life care. (NINR, 2016, para. 1)

## SUMMARY

Nursing is a practice discipline and a relatively young profession compared to the medical profession. A discipline must have a body of scientific knowledge, and for many years the nursing profession "borrowed" from other disciplines. In the past 100 years, there has been significant progress, and nursing now has its own body of knowledge and research, thanks to the work of the NINR and of nursing research journals. Although nurses conduct all types of research, in recent years there has been a greater focus on qualitative research, and currently evidence-based practice has been embraced, especially in the clinical arena.

### Further Reading

Clarke, S. (2014). The value and contribution of qualitative research to inform nurse education and policy in response to the child's experience of hospital.

*Issues in Comprehensive Pediatric Nursing, 37*(3), 153–167. doi:10.3109/01460862.2014.919366

## References

American Association of Colleges of Nursing. (2006). AACN position statement on nursing research. Retrieved from http://www.aacn.nche.edu/publications/position/nursing-research

American Association of Colleges of Nursing. (2016). AACN position statement on nursing research. Retrieved from www.aacn.org

Brink, P. J. (1979, January). Editorial. *Western Journal of Nursing Research, 1*(1), 3–4.

Carper, B. (1978). Fundamental patterns of knowing in nursing. *Advances in Nursing Science, 1*, 33–54.

Cronenwett, L., Sherwood, G., Barnsteiner, J., Disch, J., Johnson, J., Mitchell, P., . . . Warren, J. (2007). Quality and safety education for nurses. *Nursing Outlook, 55*(3), 122–131.

Eastbrooks, C. (2004). Thoughts on evidence-based nursing and its science: A Canadian perspective. *Worldviews on Evidence-Based Nursing, 1*(2), 88–91.

Fealy, G., Kelly, J., & Watson, R. (2013). Legitimacy in legacy: A discussion paper of historical scholarship published in the *Journal of Advanced Nursing*, 1976–2011. *Journal of Advanced Nursing, 69*(8), 1881–1894. doi:10.1111/jan.12048

Grove, S. K., Gray, J. R., & Burns, N. (2014). *Understanding nursing research: Building an evidence-based practice* (6th ed.). New York, NY: Elsevier.

Hunt, D. D. (2015). Understanding nursing research. Advance for Nurses. Retrieved from http://nursing.advanceweb.com/Continuing-Education/CE-Articles/Understanding-Nursing-Research.aspx

Institute of Medicine. (2010). *The future of nursing: Leading change, advancing health*. Washington, DC: National Academies Press.

Kukkala, I., & Munnukka, T. (1994). Nursing research: On what basis? *Journal of Advanced Nursing, 19*(2), 320–327. doi:10.1111/1365-2648.1994.tb01087.x

Morse, J. M. (1991). Getting started: Labels, camps, and teams. *Qualitative Health Research, 1*(1), 3–5.

National Institute of Nursing Research. (n.d.). History. Retrieved from https://www.ninr.nih.gov/aboutninr/history#.VO9lKbPF84Q

National Institute of Nursing Research. (2014, September). Grant development and management resources. Retrieved from https://www.ninr.nih.gov/researchandfunding/grant-development-and-management-resources

National Institute of Nursing Research. (2016). Mission & strategic plan. Retrieved from https://www.ninr.nih.gov/aboutninr/ninr-mission-and-strategic-plan

*Nursing Research* staff. (1952, June). Introduction to: Nursing research. *Nursing Research, 1*(1), 4.

Sarkas, J. M., & Connors, V. L. (1986). Nursing research: Historical background and teaching information strategies. *Bulletin of the Medical Library Association*, *74*(2), 121–125.

University of Maryland School of Nursing. (n.d.-a). Research at the School of Nursing. Retrieved from https://www.nursing.umaryland.edu/about/community/museum/virtual-tour/history-research/research

University of Maryland School of Nursing. (n.d.-b). The roots of nursing research. Retrieved from https://www.nursing.umaryland.edu/about/community/museum/virtual-tour/history-research/roots-research

# 13

# Professional Organizations and Key Developments

*As a nurse, we have the opportunity to heal the heart, mind, soul and body of our patients, their families and ourselves. They may forget your name, but they will never forget how you made them feel.*

—Maya Angelou

Professional organizations contribute to the development and advancement of a discipline, and throughout the past 100 years, new organizations have been created. Today, nursing is replete with organizations that represent a wide array of interests and specialties. These organizations, although created at different times with different missions and goals, must share the common goal of advancing the profession through education, research, policy, practice, and networking. Two professional organizations were created in the late 19th century in the United States. The National League for Nursing (NLN), which was originally known as the American Society of Superintendents of Training Schools for Nurses, was founded in 1893 (NLN, n.d.). The American Nurses Association (ANA) was created in 1911 and, from 1896 to 1911, was known as the Nurses Associated Alumnae for the United States and Canada (Matthews, 2012).

**In this chapter, you will learn:**

- What the following organizations are and their influence on the nursing profession:
  - National League for Nursing
  - International Council of Nurses
  - American Nurses Association
  - Sigma Theta Tau International Honor Society of Nursing
  - National Student Nurses Association
  - American Nurse Foundation
  - American Association of Colleges of Nursing
  - American Academy of Nursing
  - National Council of State Boards of Nursing
  - American Association for the History of Nursing

The historical development of professional organizations in nursing can be linked to other events that have occurred in the past 100-plus years: advancements in nursing education, both world wars, public health issues, increased workforce, greater focus on research, and a cadre of influential nurse leaders. Certainly, the nursing profession, which is 3 million strong in the United States and approximately 19 million globally (Hunt, 2014), realized significant growth and specialization at the beginning of the 21st century. Today, there are more than 100 U.S. organizations in addition to multiple international nursing organizations (Matthews, 2012). "The goal of professional organizations is to support nurses, through various elements, to evolve and lead in their everyday activities" (Schroeder, 2013, p. 99). Membership in at least one professional organization is recommended, and there is a variety of organizations from which to choose, with virtually every specialty having its own organization. Dues are paid annually, which often include discounted rates at conferences and continuing education offerings in addition to a monthly or bimonthly journal. Some organizations offer an institutional membership and reduced rates for students and retirees. Although there are too many to include in this chapter, some of the most well known and influential ones will be highlighted.

## NATIONAL LEAGUE FOR NURSING

The NLN has been in existence for more than 100 years and comprises 40,000 individual and 1,200 institutional members representing all types of nursing programs (LPN through doctorate). According to its website, the NLN (n.d.) advances the field of nursing education through professional development, research, student exam services, nurse educator certification, public policy development, and networking. A separate branch, the Accreditation Commission for Education in Nursing (ACEN), "supports the interests of nursing education, nursing practice, and the public by the functions of accreditation" (2013, para. 1). The ACEN is the oldest nursing education accreditor in existence. The accreditation process requires programs to demonstrate how they achieve the accreditation standards, whether the programs achieve their stated outcomes, and the overall quality of the program (Story et al., 2010).

## INTERNATIONAL COUNCIL OF NURSES

The International Council of Nurses (ICN) was founded in 1899 by Ethel Gordon Mason, who was a British nurse and suffragist. The focus of this international group, which originally comprised nursing leaders from North America and Europe, was to improve health and represent the interests of women and the professional image of nurses (Boschma, 2014). The mission of the ICN (2015) is "to represent nursing worldwide, advancing the profession and influencing health policy" (para. 1). The ICN developed an International Code of Ethics in 1953, with the most recent update in 2012 (ICN, 2015). "The ICN Code of Ethics guides nurses in everyday choices and it supports their refusal to participate in activities that conflict with caring and healing" (ICN, 2012, para. 3). Today, the ICN continues to focus on nursing issues with an overall goal of promoting health of individuals, populations, and societies (ICN, 2015).

## AMERICAN NURSES ASSOCIATION

The ANA has operated since 1896 and represents 3.6 million professional nurses in the United States (ANA, n.d., 2016b). The ANA has been very influential over the past century and has developed myriad initiatives (see Exhibit 13.1). For example, the ANA developed nursing's code of ethics, which serves as a guide to practice (ANA, n.d.).

Exhibit 13.1

### Timeline of ANA Initiatives (ANA, n.d.)

**1901**—"The first state nurses' associations were organized to work toward state laws to control nursing practice" (p. 1).

**1914**—"ANA established the Central Information Bureau for Legislation and Information to supply data concerning the work of state boards of nurse examiners" (p. 5).

**1922**—"ANA increased its dues from 15 cents to 50 cents per member to undertake the financial responsibility of maintaining a national headquarters" (p. 7).

**1926**—The ANA amended its bylaws to state that to be a member one has to be a registered nurse.

**1938**—"ANA recommended a salary schedule for nurses comparable to those of other women workers, a 48-hour week for nurses practicing in institutions, and vacations with pay" (p. 12).

**1950**—"ANA adopted a code of ethics for professional nursing" (p. 17).

**1973**—The American Academy of Nursing was created "with the adoption of a resolution by the ANA Board of Directors, which designated thirty-six charter fellows, named pro tem officers, and directed that specific action be taken to establish the academy" (p. 29).

**1991**—The ANA created the American Nurse Credentialing Center.

**2006**—A new official journal of the ANA was launched, *American Nurse Today,* in October.

**2008**—"The ANA Board of Directors endorsed the document, 'Consensus Model for APRN Regulations: Licensure, Accreditation, Certification and Education'" (p. 53).

**2013**—"ANA spearheaded an effort to develop national, interdisciplinary, safe patient handling and mobility (SPHM) standards to be applicable across the care continuum" (p. 60).

The ANA (2016a) also shapes and supports health care policy, including the Registered Nurse Safe Staffing Act and the Nurse and Health Care Worker Protection Act.

**Fast Facts in a Nutshell**

On August 25, 1908, the National Association of Colored Graduate Nurses was founded when 52 African American nurses gathered in New York City. The group focused on eliminating discrimination and developing leadership among African American nurses. In 1951, it became part of the ANA (n.d.).

## SIGMA THETA TAU INTERNATIONAL HONOR SOCIETY OF NURSING

The Sigma Theta Tau International Honor Society of Nursing was founded in 1922 by six nurses at the Indiana University Training School for Nurses. Today, there are approximately 500 chapters and 135,000 members in more than 90 countries. Student nurses who meet the criteria are invited to join, and nurse leaders may apply. "The mission of the Honor Society of Nursing, Sigma Theta Tau International, is advancing world health and celebrating nursing excellence in scholarship, leadership, and service" (Sigma Theta Tau International, 2016c, para. 1). The honor society became the first organization in the United States to fund nursing research in 1936 and now with its partners raises more than $200,000 per year for nursing research (Sigma Theta Tau International, 2016c).

### Fast Facts in a Nutshell

The founders chose the name Sigma Theta Tau from the Greek words *storgé, tharsos,* and *timé,* meaning "love," "courage," and "honor" (Sigma Theta Tau International, 2016c).

## NATIONAL STUDENT NURSES ASSOCIATION

The National Student Nurses Association was founded in 1952 to mentor students and foster professional development in nursing students. Today, there are more than 60,000 members in all 50 states in addition to Puerto Rico, Guam, and the U.S. Virgin Islands. The National Student Nurses Association (2016) holds a yearly convention, and student representatives from the various schools attend.

## AMERICAN NURSES FOUNDATION

The American Nurses Foundation was founded in 1955 to complement the work of the ANA with a focus on charitable contributions, research, and education. Its mission "is to transform the health of the nation through the power of nursing" (American Nurses Foundation, n.d., para. 1).

## AMERICAN ASSOCIATION OF COLLEGES OF NURSING

The American Association of Colleges of Nursing was established in 1969 to advance nursing education at the undergraduate and graduate levels. According to its website, it remains the only national organization dedicated exclusively to meeting this goal. Throughout the years, it has developed various initiatives and provides various educational offerings and conferences. The American Association of Colleges of Nursing plays an important role in nursing and health care policy. There is also an accrediting branch, the Commission on Collegiate Nursing Education, that serves as the accrediting body for many undergraduate and graduate programs (American Association of Colleges of Nursing, 2017).

## AMERICAN ACADEMY OF NURSING

The American Academy of Nursing falls under the corporate sponsorship of the ANA and held its first meeting in 1973. The academy serves the public and the nursing profession by advancing health policy and practice through the generation, synthesis, and dissemination of nursing knowledge. The academy has 2,400 members, who are known as "Fellows" and have been invited to join based on their significant contribution to nursing. They are also expected to continue to play a vital role in shaping nursing and health care (American Academy of Nursing, 2015).

## NATIONAL COUNCIL OF STATE BOARDS OF NURSING

The National Council of State Boards of Nursing is an independent organization that was founded in 1978 and serves as a unifying body of the individual state boards of nursing, enabling them to collaborate on matters of common interest, such as the development of nursing licensure exams and public health, safety, and welfare. It also develops the National Council Licensure Examination (NCLEX) test plan and examination and in 1994 began offering the NCLEX using computerized adaptive testing (National Council of State Boards of Nursing, 2017). Prior to 1982, graduate nurses took the test over 2 days, and it had five separate exams: medical nursing, surgical nursing, pediatric nursing, maternity nursing, and psychiatric nursing (National Council of State Boards of Nursing, 2014).

## AMERICAN ASSOCIATION FOR THE HISTORY OF NURSES

The American Association for the History of Nurses, which was originally called the International History of Nursing Society, was founded in 1978. The purpose of the association is to "foster the importance of history as relevant to understanding the past, defining the present, and influencing the future of nursing" (American Association for the History of Nurses, 2007, para. 1). The mission is to advance historical scholarship in health care and nursing and promote historians' development (American Association for the History of Nurses, 2007). (See the interview with Jean Whelan in this book's introduction for more information on this organization.)

## PROFESSIONAL ORGANIZATIONS AROUND THE GLOBE

The ICN is an organization that includes nurses from around the world. In addition, many countries have their own professional organizations similar to the ones in the United States. For example, in England, there is the Royal College of Nursing, the Foundation of Nursing Studies, and the Florence Nightingale Foundation. France has the French Nursing Research Association, and Ireland has the Nursing Board of Ireland and the National Council for the Professional Development of Nursing and Midwifery. The European Union has several professional organizations, including the European Honour Society of Nursing and Midwifery. According to Sigma Theta Tau International (2016a, 2016b), there are 29 professional organizations in Africa, such as the Ghana Registered Nurses Association, and there are 27 professional organizations in the Asia/Pacific region, including three in Hong Kong alone. Six continents have nursing organizations.

## SUMMARY

Professional nursing organizations have been in existence since the late 1800s and have had a major influence on nurses, the nursing profession, and health care. Currently, there are organizations in many countries for virtually every specialty, and they all offer something unique to their members. This chapter highlighted some of the significant and influential professional organizations.

## References


Accreditation Commission for Education in Nursing. (2013). Mission | purpose | goals. Retrieved from http://www.acenursing.org/mission-purpose-goals/

American Academy of Nursing. (2015). About the Academy. Retrieved from http://www.aannet.org/about/about-the-academy

American Association of Colleges of Nursing (2017). About AACN. Retrieved from http://www.aacn.nche.edu/about-aacn

American Association for the History of Nurses. (2007). About AAHN. Retrieved from https://www.aahn.org/about.html

American Nurses Association. (n.d.). Historical review. Retrieved from http://www.nursingworld.org/FunctionalMenuCategories/AboutANA/History/BasicHistoricalReview.pdf

American Nurses Association. (2016a). 2015 annual report. Retrieved from http://www.nursingworld.org/FunctionalMenuCategories/AboutANA/Annual-Reports/Annual-Report-2015.pdf

American Nurses Association. (2016b). About ANA. Retrieved from http://www.nursingworld.org/FunctionalMenuCategories/AboutANA

American Nurses Foundation. (n.d.). History. Retrieved from http://www.anfonline.org/Main/AboutANF/History

Boschma, G. (2014). International nursing history: The International Council of Nurses history collective and beyond. *Nursing History Review, 22,* 114–118.

Hunt, D. (2014). *The nurse professional: Leveraging your education for transition into practice.* New York, NY: Springer Publishing.

International Council of Nurses. (2012). *The ICN code of ethics for nurses.* Retrieved from http://www.icn.ch/who-we-are/code-of-ethics-for-nurses

International Council of Nurses. (2015, April). Our mission, strategic intent, core values, and priorities. Retrieved from http://www.icn.ch/who-we-are/our-mission-strategic-intent-core-values-and-priorities

Matthews, J. (2012). Role of professional organizations in advocating for the nursing profession. *OJIN: The Online Journal of Issues in Nursing, 17*(1). doi:10.3912/OJIN.Vol17No01Man03

National Council of State Boards of Nursing. (2014). Pencils down, booklets closed. *In Focus, 1*(2), 10–16.

National Council of State Boards of Nursing. (2017). History. Retrieved from http://www.ncsbn.org/ history.htm

National League for Nursing. (n.d.). Overview. Retrieved from http://www.nln.org/about

National Student Nurses Association. (2016). About us. Retrieved from http://www.nsna.org/about-nsna.html

Schroeder, R. T. (2013). The value of belonging to a professional nursing organization. *AORN Journal, 98*(2), 99–101. doi:10.1016/j.aorn.2013.06

Sigma Theta Tau International Honor Society of America. (2016a). Africa nursing organizations. Retrieved from http://www.nursingsociety.org/connect-engage/our-global-impact/professional-nursing-organizations/africa-nursing-organizations

Sigma Theta Tau International Honor Society of America. (2016b). Asia/Pacific nursing organizations. Retrieved from http://www.nursingsociety.org/connect-engage/our-global-impact/professional-nursing-organizations/asia-pacific-nursing-organizations

Sigma Theta Tau International Honor Society of America. (2016c). STTI organizational fact sheet. Retrieved from http://www.nursingsociety.org/connect-engage/about-stti/sigma-theta-tau-international-organizational-fact-sheet

Story, L., Butts, J., Bishop, S., Green, L., Johnson, K., & Mattison, H. (2010). Innovative strategies for nursing education program evaluation. *Journal of Nursing Education*, *49*(6), 351–354. doi:10.3928/01484834-20100217-07

# 14

# The Nurse of Tomorrow

*Do not go where the path may lead, go instead where there is no path and leave a trail.*

—Ralph Waldo Emerson

History is always fluid, and the history of nursing and health care is evolving rapidly, with developments in science and technology, increased awareness of the importance of global health, and the quest to provide safe, effective, high-quality care. Scientific advancements continue to promise new health care technology and cures, and although there is always uncertainty regarding the future, the foundations have been laid to continue to improve health and health care well into the 21st century. In the recent past, the major driving forces in health care have been the Affordable Care Act, the Institute of Medicine's report on the future of nursing, technology, genomics, and global health.

**In this chapter, you will learn:**

- The significance of the Institute of Medicine's report *The Future of Nursing*
- Current health policy issues
- Key effects of the Affordable Care Act
- How advances in technology and genomics affect nursing care
- Current global health initiatives

The new millennium was awaited with bated breath and excitement, as well as fears of what would happen at the turn of a new century. Everyone was preparing for Y2K, a potential crisis in which computers worldwide would stop working properly on January 1, 2000, due to the way dates were digitally stored. This was especially true of health care organizations, which were faced with uncertainty regarding technology and whether Y2K would have a negative impact on the various information technologies used in hospitals and virtually every organization. Thankfully, the transition went smoothly. Since that time, technology has continued to advance, which for the most part has had a positive effect on nursing, medicine, and health care. The Patient Protection and Affordable Care Act (2010; ACA) was fraught with uncertainty, and although it was passed, there is still uncertainty and conflict over its merits. The nursing profession has reached new heights and has become more autonomous. Many nurses have achieved higher levels of education, which certainly has been influenced by the *Future of Nursing* report, which called for 80% of registered nurses (RNs) to earn their bachelor of science in nursing (BSN) degree by 2020 and for doubling the number of nurses with doctoral degrees (Institute of Medicine, 2010).

## THE INSTITUTE OF MEDICINE'S *FUTURE OF NURSING* REPORT

The Institute of Medicine's (2010) *Future of Nursing* report has had a profound effect on the nursing profession. It resulted from a 2-year initiative of the Robert Wood Johnson Foundation and the Institute of Medicine to evaluate and act on the need to transform nursing. The report includes four key messages and eight recommendations (Institute of Medicine, 2010). The four key messages of the report are as follows:

- Nurses should practice to the full extent of their education and training.
- Nurses should achieve higher levels of education and training through an improved education system that promotes seamless academic progression.
- Nurses should be full partners, with physicians and other health professionals, in redesigning health care in the United States.
- Effective workforce planning and policy making require better data collection and an improved information infrastructure. (Institute of Medicine, 2010, p. 29)

The recommendations were put into action by individual state action coalitions that were created for this purpose. Although each action coalition is unique, each is committed to advancing the profession and implementing the recommendations of this landmark report (*Campaign for Action,* n.d.). Notably, significant progress has been made in advancing education and expanding the scope of practice. To date, 22 states (and the District of Columbia) allow for full practice of nurse practitioners, 16 states have reduced practice, and 12 states have restricted practice (American Association of Nurse Practitioners, 2017). Seemingly, the role of the advanced practice RN will continue to expand. For example, the Veterans Administration is one organization currently considering expanding the role of the NP within its health care system (Proposed Rule—Advanced Practice Registered Nurses, 2016). The goal of increasing the number of baccalaureate-prepared nurses to be 80% of RNs by 2020 is ambitious; progress has been made, and there has been a steady increase in enrollment in entry-level, accelerated enrollment, and RN-to-BSN programs (Hudson, 2016). Another initiative is to increase the number of nurses in leadership positions; for example, the Nurses on Boards Coalition (2016) is campaigning to enhance the health of the United States and its communities by adding 10,000 nurses to boards by 2020. According to Buxton and Scott (2015), nurses were called to action due to the Affordable Care Act (ACA) and the Institute of Medicine's *Future of Nursing* report and are in a unique position to lead the interprofessional team as health care delivery models become more community based. This is just a brief overview of the report and progress on its recommendations to date. Clearly, the implementation is a work in progress, and the report will most likely continue to shape the future of nursing and health care.

## Fast Facts in a Nutshell

*The Future of Nursing* report's call to double the number of nurses with doctorate degrees was fulfilled in 2014, when there were 21,280 employed nurses with this qualification (American Community Survey, as cited in *Campaign for Action,* 2016).

## HEALTH CARE POLICY

Several policy and legislative issues are being addressed, and their outcomes will certainly shape the future of nursing. Scope-of-practice issues are being examined in multiple states. The BSN in Ten continues to be supported in New York, and in each legislative session, progress is made toward passing this bill, which would require nurses with associate degrees to earn their BSN within 10 years (Trossman, 2008).

Although there has been opposition to this type of legislation in recent years, it has become more widely embraced. Staffing ratios is another area being debated, especially in light of serious issues with quality of care and adverse medical events. The American Nurses Association (2014) predicts that due to factors such as our expanding aging population, health care reform, and the number of nurses who will retire in the next 15 to 20 years, we will experience another major shortage.

Nursing schools are forming partnerships to expand student capacity. As part of this effort, in 2010, the American Association of Colleges of Nursing (AACN) "announced the expansion of NursingCAS, the nation's centralized application service for RN programs, to include graduate nursing programs" (AACN, 2014). This identifies schools that have vacant seats to be filled and maximize the education capacity of nursing programs. In addition to this, some states are offering funding. For example, in 2014, "the University of Wisconsin (UW) announced the $3.2 million Nurses for Wisconsin initiative—funded through a UW System Economic Development Incentive Grant—to provide fellowships and loan forgiveness for future nurse faculty who agree to teach in the state after graduation" (AACN, 2015). In July 2010, the Robert Wood Johnson Foundation (RWJF) published in its newsletter, *Charting Nursing's Future*, a policy brief titled "Expanding America's Capacity to Educate Nurses." This brief describes the innovations of 12 partnerships that are effectively addressing the nursing and nurse faculty shortages. Among the policy recommendations advanced in this brief are requiring all new nurses to complete a BSN program within 10 years of licensure and providing pathways into baccalaureate and graduate programs (RWJF, 2010).

## AFFORDABLE CARE ACT

The ACA was passed to address ongoing health care needs, decrease costs, focus more on health and wellness promotion, and close the gap of individuals who were uninsured or underinsured (Patient Protection and Affordable Care Act, 2010). "The Affordable Care Act was passed by Congress and then signed into law by the President on March 23, 2010. On June 28, 2012, the Supreme Court rendered a final decision to uphold the health care law" (American Library Association, 2014, para. 1). The law is more than 950 pages long (Patient Protection and Affordable Care Act, 2010), and there are proponents and opponents of this act. With the new president, there is some uncertainty regarding the staying power of the ACA because in general, the Democrats support the act, whereas the Republicans do not support it.

Lacey (2015) breaks down key points of the ACA and its effect on nursing. She posits that since the passing of the ACA, more than 9 million have been insured with expectations of an additional 30 million over the next 5 to 10 years, placing an additional strain on an already tight nursing market. Because preexisting conditions are covered, more nurses will be needed to provide complex care. Payment models and quality-of-care initiatives will also require nurses to be proactive. She calls on all nurses to create new solutions for the complexity of our health care system and the health of our nation.

## ADVANCES IN TECHNOLOGY

Technology has grown exponentially in recent years and will most likely continue on this path of rapid expansion, thus continually changing the face of nursing, medicine, and health care. Technology has had a significant impact around the world, not only in health care but also in many other areas. With regard to nursing, technology has affected many aspects of care and is intended to assist nurses in the provision of safe, effective, quality care. It is important to remember that technology is a tool and still subject to user error, but it has the potential to greatly improve health care (Piscotty, Kalisch, & Gracey-Thomas, 2015). Current technology available in health care organizations includes the following:

- Electronic health records
- All types of medical equipment
- Smartphones and various apps
- Robotics
- Telehealth
- Remote monitoring
- Three-dimensional printing

**Fast Facts in a Nutshell**

Bar coding has decreased medication errors by 80% (Foote & Coleman, 2008).

## GENOMICS AND DISEASE MANAGEMENT

*Genomics* has been defined in the following way: "Genomics is the science that aims to decipher and understand the entire genetic information of an organism . . . encoded in DNA and corresponding complements. . . . Experts in genomics strive to determine complete DNA sequences and perform genetic mapping to help understand disease" (Elsersawi, 2016, Glossary section). Currently, genomics is being used to screen and diagnose, identify at-risk individuals, and optimize drug therapy benefits (Calzone et al., 2013). According to Calzone and colleagues (2010), "Nurses must be competent in genomics to provide safe, cost-effective, quality health care" (as cited in Calzone et al., 2013, p. 97), especially because genomics is constantly changing. As advances continue, it will be important for nurses to have continuing education in genomics.

**Fast Facts in a Nutshell**

"All aspects of the healthcare continuum are influenced by genomic developments. As such, the use of genomic information and technology is no longer dependent on referral to a genetic specialist, but has transitioned into nonspecialty healthcare delivery" (Calzone et al., 2013, p. 97).

## GLOBAL HEALTH

Global health has taken on greater significance in recent years, and nurses continue to play a key role. In 2014, a Global Advisory Panel on the Future of Nursing & Midwifery (2016) was created by the Sigma Theta Tau International Honor Society of Nursing. The purpose of this

Exhibit 14.1

**The United Nations (2015) Millennium Development Goals**

- Eradicate extreme hunger and poverty
- Achieve universal primary education
- Promote gender equality and empower women
- Reduce child mortality
- Improve maternal health
- Combat HIV/AIDS, malaria, and other diseases
- Ensure environmental sustainability
- Promote global partnership for development (para. 1)

panel is to support and improve global health around the world and to address the United Nations (2015) Millennium Development Goals (see Exhibit 14.1). The goals of the panel include the following:

- Facilitate, now and in the future, conversation about top issues related to global health, nursing, and midwifery.
- Advance global health by aligning social, environmental, and economic pathways.
- Determine how nursing and midwifery can take the initiative in the alignment (Global Advisory Panel on the Future of Nursing & Midwifery, 2016).

Global issues are constantly changing with the advent of various communicable diseases such as Ebola and the Zika virus. Both natural and manmade disasters continue to occur at an alarming rate, which further highlights the need for a highly skilled and educated workforce (Centers for Disease Control and Prevention [CDC], 2016; Hageman et al., 2016).

## SUMMARY

History is in the making in nursing. This chapter highlighted some of the driving forces in the changes that have taken place since the new millennium and the possible direction in which we will move. Because history is fluid and external and internal forces are constantly changing, we must be prepared to guide our profession into the future.

## References


American Association of Colleges of Nursing. (2014). Nursing shortage fact sheet. Retrieved from http://www.aacn.nche.edu/media-relations/NrsgShortageFS.pdf

American Association of Colleges of Nursing. (2015). Nursing faculty shortage. Retrieved from http://www.aacn.nche.edu/media-relations/fact-sheets/nursing-faculty-shortage

American Association of Nurse Practitioners. (2017). State practice environment. Retrieved from https://www.aanp.org/legislation-regulation/state-legislation/state-practice-environment

American Library Association. (2014). Affordable Care Act. Retrieved from http://www.ala.org/tools/atoz/affordable-care-act

American Nurses Association. (2014, April). Nursing shortage. Retrieved from http://www.aacn.nche.edu/media-relations/fact-sheets/nursing-shortage

Buxton, T., & Scott, D. (2015). The Affordable Care Act and 21st-century nursing: Are you ready? *Colorado Nurse, 115*(3), 15.

Calzone, K. A., Jenkins, J., Bakos, A. D., Cashion, A. K., Donaldson, N., Feero, W. G., . . . Webb, J. A. (2013). A blueprint for genomic nursing science. *Journal of Nursing Scholarship, 45*(1), 96–104. doi:10.1111/jnu.12007

*Campaign for Action.* (n.d.). State action coalitions. Retrieved from http://campaignforaction.org/our-network/state-action-coalitions

*Campaign for Action.* (2016, May). Welcome to the future of nursing: Campaign for Action dashboard. Retrieved from https://campaignforaction.org/wp-content/uploads/2016/04/Campaign-Dashboard-5-19-16.pdf

Centers for Disease Control and Prevention. (2016). CDC and OSHA issue interim guidance for protecting workers from occupational exposure to Zika virus. Retrieved from https://www.cdc.gov/media/releases/2016/s0422-interim-guidance-zika.html

Elsersawi, A. (2016). *Genes mapping, epigenetics, cloning therapy.* Bloomington, IN: AuthorHouse.

Foote, S., & Coleman, J. (2008). Success story. Medication administration: The implementation process of bar-coding for medication administration to enhance medication safety. *Nursing Economics, 26*(3), 207–210.

Global Advisory Panel on the Future of Nursing & Midwifery. (2016). The Global Advisory Panel on the Future of Nursing & Midwifery. Retrieved from http://www.gapfon.org

Hageman, J. C., Hazim, C., Wilson, K., Malpiedi, P., Gupta, N., Bennett, S., . . . & Park, B. J. (2016). Infection prevention and control for Ebola in health care settings—West Africa and United States. *Morbidity and Mortality Weekly Report, 65*(Suppl. 3), 50–56. doi:10.15585/mmwr.su6503a8

Hudson, L. R. (2016). Assessing the report: Has the future of nursing been impacted? *Iowa Board of Nursing Newsletter, 35*(1), 1–2.

Institute of Medicine. (2010). *The future of nursing: Leading change, advancing health.* Washington, DC: National Academies Press.

Lacey, S. (2015). The Affordable Care Act (ACA) upheld: What's next for staff nurses, nursing leaders and the profession? *Mississippi RN, 77*(4), 4.

Nurses on Boards Coalition. (2016). Nurses on Boards Coalition. Retrieved from http://www.nursesonboardscoalition.org

Patient Protection and Affordable Care Act, 42 U.S.C. § 18001 (2010).

Piscotty, R. J., Jr., Kalisch, B., & Gracey-Thomas, A. (2015). Impact of healthcare information technology on nursing practice. *Journal of Nursing Scholarship, 47*(4), 287–293. doi:10.1111/jnu.12138

Proposed Rule—Advanced Practice Registered Nurses, 81 Fed. Reg. 33155 (proposed May 25, 2016) (to be codified as 38 C.F.R. pt. 17).

Robert Wood Johnson Foundation. (2010). Expanding America's capacity to educate nurses: Diverse, state-level partnerships are creating promising models and results. Retrieved from http://www.rwjf.org/content/dam/farm/reports/issue_briefs/2010/rwjf61023

Trossman, S. (2008). BSN in ten. *Inside ANA, 3*(11). Retrieved from https://www.americannursetoday.com/bsn-in-ten

United Nations. (2015). News on millennium development goals. Retrieved from http://www.un.org/millenniumgoals

# Index